The Krebiozen Hoax

The Krebiozen Hoax

How a Mysterious Cancer Drug Shook Organized Medicine

MATTHEW C. EHRLICH

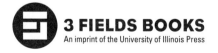

3 FIELDS BOOKS
An imprint of the University of Illinois Press

3 Fields Books is an imprint of the University of Illinois Press.
© 2024 by the Board of Trustees
of the University of Illinois
All rights reserved
Manufactured in the United States of America
1 2 3 4 5 C P 5 4 3 2 1
∞ This book is printed on acid-free paper.

Library of Congress Cataloging-in-Publication Data
Names: Ehrlich, Matthew C., 1962– author.
Title: The Krebiozen hoax : how a mysterious cancer drug shook
    organized medicine / Matthew C. Ehrlich.
Description: Urbana : 3 Fields books, an imprint of the University
    of Illinois Press, [2024] | Includes bibliographical references and
    index.
Identifiers: LCCN 2024002511 (print) | LCCN 2024002512
    (ebook) | ISBN 9780252046018 (cloth ; alk. paper) |
    ISBN 9780252088117 (paperback ; alk. paper) | ISBN
    9780252047190 (ebook)
Subjects: MESH: Ivy, A. C. (Andrew Conway), 1893–1978. |
    University of Illinois Chicago Professional Colleges. | University
    of Illinois (Urbana-Champaign campus). | Neoplasms—drug
    therapy | Neoplasms—history | Creatinine—therapeutic use |
    Quackery—history | Fraud—history | History, 20th Century |
    Illinois
Classification: LCC RC271.C5 (print) | LCC RC271.C5 (ebook) |
    NLM QZ 267 | DDC 616.99/4061—dc23/eng/20240214
LC record available at https://lccn.loc.gov/2024002511
LC ebook record available at https://lccn.loc.gov/2024002512

Contents

Acknowledgments

My appreciation goes to the staffs of multiple archives for providing generous amounts of time and assistance, sometimes under challenging pandemic-related conditions. Thanks to William Maher, Joanne Kaczmarek, Linda Stepp, Ellen Swain, Jameatris Rimkus, Katie Nichols, Sammi Merritt, Will Doty, and the rest of the staff of the University of Illinois at Urbana-Champaign (UIUC) Archives. Thanks also to Sarah Bial and the staff of the History, Philosophy, and Newspaper Library at UIUC, as well as to Ann Panthen and the staff of the Champaign County Historical Archives at the Urbana Free Library in Illinois. In Chicago, thanks to Jorie Braunold, Kelsey Walsh, and the staff of the American Medical Association Archives; to Laura Mills and the staff of the Roosevelt University Archives; to Ellen Keith and the staff of the Abakanowicz Research Center at the Chicago History Museum; and to Leanna Barcelona and the staff of the University of Illinois-Chicago Archives. Thanks as well to Kolter Campbell and the staff of the McCormick Library of Special Collections and University Archives at Northwestern University in Evanston, Illinois.

In Austin, Texas, thanks to Brian McNerney, Jenna De Graffenried, and the rest of the staff of the Lyndon Baines Johnson Presidential Library and Museum; as well as to Amy Wagner, Cristina Meisner, Kathryn Millan, and the rest of the staff of the Harry Ransom Center at the University of Texas. In College Park, Maryland, thanks to Tom McAnear and the staff of the National Archives and Records Administration. In Laramie, Wyoming, thanks to Vicki Lynne Glantz and the staff of the American Heritage Center at the University of Wyoming. At the Food and Drug Administration, thanks to Vanessa Burrows for assistance with research and images, as well as to Kim Morris for responding to Freedom of Information Act requests.

In Boston, thanks to Stacey Chandler for responding to queries on holdings in the John F. Kennedy Presidential Library and Museum Archives.

My thanks to Martha Bayne at the University of Illinois Press (UIP) for expressing interest in this project and shepherding it to completion with help from UIP's Mariah Schaefer. Thanks as well to press director Laurie Matheson, editor-in-chief Daniel Nasset, and the rest of the UIP staff, including Angela Burton, Kevin Cunningham, Jennie Fisher, Heather Gernenz, Dustin Hubbart, Tad Ringo, Michael Roux, Roberta Sparenberg, and Kristina Stonehill. The UIP Faculty Board, John Thelin, William London, and two anonymous reviewers provided helpful feedback on drafts of this manuscript. Tony Dudek at Tribune Content Agency in Chicago and Colleen Layton at the Chicago History Museum assisted in obtaining images. Geof Garvey copyedited the final manuscript.

Finally, my love and thanks to my family, including my late father George Ehrlich and my late aunt Martha Ehrlich Mlinarich, both of whom were raised in Chicago and were proud University of Illinois alumni.

The Krebiozen Hoax

INTRODUCTION

Cancer, Quackery, and Hope

There once was a drug named Krebiozen;
It came from below the horizon.
It used to be said, by patients now dead,
Now what do we put our reliance on?
—Limerick attributed to University of Illinois
president George Stoddard and University
of Illinois provost Coleman Griffith, both of
whom would lose their jobs over Krebiozen[1]

On March 26, 1951, one of America's most respected scientists called a meeting at Chicago's Drake Hotel to make a dramatic announcement: he and a Yugoslavian refugee doctor had found a drug that showed great promise in treating cancer. The scientist was Andrew Ivy, vice president of the University of Illinois (U of I) and designated spokesperson for medical ethics at the Nazi war crimes trials in Nuremberg. *Time* magazine had gone as far as to pronounce him "the conscience of U.S. science." Ivy's Yugoslavian collaborator was Stevan Durovic, said to have discovered the new drug in Argentina after the Nazis forced him to flee his homeland. The drug itself was called Krebiozen, a name that was supposed to connote "cancer suppressor" or "regulator of growth."[2]

Krebiozen's unveiling electrified people around the world. Cancer sufferers and their loved ones deluged the U of I with thousands of calls and messages begging for the drug. One doctor opined that "Krebiozen may be one of the greatest, if not the greatest" discoveries in medical history.[3] But other representatives of organized medicine were immediately suspicious.

Virtually none of them had ever heard of Stevan Durovic or his brother Marko, who had followed Stevan to Chicago to promote Krebiozen. Stevan had never published in a scientific journal. The Durovics refused to reveal even to Andrew Ivy precisely how the drug was made, other than that it involved stimulating the immune systems of horses and extracting their blood. Rather than using the conventional means of announcing a new scientific discovery—through academic venues subject to rigorous peer review—Ivy had staged the equivalent of a product launch, inviting prominent politicians from Chicago and downstate Illinois along with wealthy benefactors and members of the press. Moreover, although Ivy denied any advance knowledge of it, that meeting had been promoted through a sensational news release: "The battle of medical science to find a cure for cancer achieved its realization today."[4] Within months, the American Medical Association (AMA) announced that its review of patient case histories had shown Krebiozen to be worthless; later, U of I president George Stoddard asserted that there was no such thing as Krebiozen.

Ivy and the Durovics fought back. They accused the AMA of conspiring with powerful business interests to kill Krebiozen after failing to seize control of it. Illinois lawmakers, some of whom despised Stoddard because of his liberalism and seeming highhandedness, began a lengthy set of hearings on the conspiracy charges and the state university's possible complicity in suppressing the drug. Stoddard and U of I provost Coleman Griffith were ousted from their administrative posts. In the following years, the controversy spread beyond Illinois as groups formed across the country championing Krebiozen. Movie star Gloria Swanson raised money for the drug; environmentalist Rachel Carson took the medicine to try to fight her cancer. Pro-Krebiozen demonstrators (some wearing badges saying, "I need Krebiozen to live!") were arrested outside the White House and bodily hauled out of federal offices. Along with members of Congress, they lobbied fiercely for what they called a "fair test" of the drug. Nevertheless, the Food and Drug Administration (FDA), which had just been granted expanded powers, declared that Krebiozen did nothing to stop cancer. Ivy and the Durovics were indicted on charges of defrauding people who had paid nearly ten dollars per ampule of the drug. After a nine-month trial in Chicago that ended in early 1966, the defendants were acquitted, with the verdicts tainted by accusations of jury tampering. Then Krebiozen sank back below the horizon, to be replaced by other unproven remedies purported to treat cancer and other medical ills.

This book resurrects Krebiozen's improbable story, rife with equal parts intrigue and farce, hubris and pathos. The story represents a significant episode in the history of Illinois, exposing political rifts and machinations extending from Chicago to the rest of the state; it also is a significant episode in the history of the state's flagship university, which was then at the forefront of dramatic changes in American higher education. Beyond that, Krebiozen highlights a key historical moment for the FDA, as the agency exerted new regulatory muscle and subsequently experienced a backlash against the perceived overreach of the medical establishment. Finally, Krebiozen is a quintessential example of quackery, reflecting broad, longstanding divisions in American life. It foreshadowed today's bitter debates over health misinformation, medical freedom, and scientific and educational expertise.

• • •

Proponents of evidence-based science and medicine often find themselves on the defensive these days. "A new legion of social media 'experts,' indifferent to established facts, supply a rapt mass audience all manner of crackpot opinions about Covid, cancer, autism, vaccines, vitamins, immune-boosters, anti-ageing remedies, chelation and detoxification," one scientist has written. He excoriates "celebrity public health menaces" who "peddle nostrums and elixirs of no value," as well as politicians who "mangle and censor science in public health messages and policies."[5] The COVID-19 pandemic exacerbated worries about health misinformation. Proponents of alleged COVID remedies including ivermectin and hydroxychloroquine were blamed for encouraging individuals to shun more effective therapies, even in some cases at the cost of their own lives. Nor is the reliance on such remedies a recent development. One medical researcher asserts that phony COVID treatments are "no different than quackery going back centuries," while also noting that purveyors of COVID misinformation have copied tactics long employed by cancer quacks.[6]

Quackery has in fact been a perennial feature of the American scene, as has fraud generally. "Since the earliest years of American independence, the most prevalent business frauds have occurred over and over again, even if dressed up in different garb or framed in newfangled terms," writes historian Edward J. Balleisen. He says that charlatans have thrived in a culture that has been devoted to "lionization of entrepreneurial freedom" and to the promise of making a fast buck. Quackery, however—the promotion of supposedly miraculous medical devices and therapies that do not actually work—preys on more than just greed. In the words of Gary and Linda Friedlaender, "the uncertainties of illness and the mysteries of death, coupled with the instinct and the passion to survive, create a natural human vulnerability in which patients tend to believe what is comforting and hopeful."[7] That vulnerability has been exploited by fraudsters brimming with avarice, self-delusion, or both. Their ranks have ranged from John Brinkley, who in the first decades of the twentieth century falsely promised to restore men's virility by transplanting goat testicles into them; to Elizabeth Holmes, who in the first decades of the twenty-first century falsely promised to provide early detection of a multitude of diseases through a mere prick of a person's finger.[8]

Cancer in particular has attracted a long line of promoters of unproven and fraudulent treatments that have drawn the ire of organized medicine. Norman Baker peddled a grasses-and-herbs remedy; Harry Hoxsey boosted a therapy of herbs and caustic pastes; William Frederick Koch hawked his "Glyoxylide" formula. After Krebiozen faded from public view, Laetrile garnered widespread popular and political support in the 1970s. The medicine, which was derived from fruit kernels, was legalized in many US states before controlled clinical trials found it to be ineffective in treating cancer and potentially dangerous to its users. During that same period, Nobel laureate Linus Pauling championed vitamin C as a cancer therapy. When clinical trials repudiated Pauling's claims, he charged that the trials had been biased and fraudulent. And so it has continued: a list of unproven and disproven cancer treatments includes nearly 150 such remedies, ranging from aromatherapy, light therapy, and magnetic therapy to coffee enemas, emu oil, and urine.[9]

What are the typical characteristics of medical quackery, and why does it persist so stubbornly? Nina Shapiro observes that "today there is more wizardry and trickery in the health sphere than almost everywhere else," enabled by the ready accessibility of online health information and misinformation. In such a climate, quackery's "tricks of the trade" become even more widely used. Those tricks are nothing new; just as is true of business frauds, quackery tends to repeat the same traits and patterns over the years.[10]

James Harvey Young, the foremost historian of quackery, listed ten such traits. *Exploitation of fear* implies that many mainstream health therapies are "essentially useless and more painful than the disease itself," whereas unproven remedies offer the *promise of painless treatment and good results* while also making *claims of a miraculous scientific breakthrough*. Although mainstream doctors and scientists have argued that cancer is not one disease but many related diseases with potentially different causes, quacks promote *one cause: one therapeutic system* panaceas. They use *the Galileo ploy* by contending that their "maligners are wrong, just as earlier critics condemned pioneering explorers, inventors, and scientists," such as Galileo (even though in reality scientific and medical breakthroughs rarely are achieved by heroic individuals working in isolation). Quacks also advance a *conspiracy theory* insinuating that their ill-intentioned enemies are in league against them. They make *shifts to adjust to circumstances* "if some change might offer greater prosperity or safety," and they display a *reliance on testimonials* to bolster their claims. Those claims represent a *distortion of the idea of freedom,* the implication being that people have a fundamental right to try even ineffective or dangerous remedies. Finally, quackery typically involves *large sums of money* being separated from victims by the quacks.[11]

Although Young based his list on multiple examples of quackery during the nineteenth and twentieth centuries, medical fraud in our own times displays similar characteristics. For example, Elizabeth Holmes was said to view herself as a contemporary Marie Curie who ultimately would be vindicated in the face of her doubters, a variation of the Galileo ploy. The diagnostic system that her Theranos company promoted was supposed to revolutionize health care by offering a cheap, painless, and more effective alternative to standard blood draws that relied on fearsome needles. Theranos said that the technology that supposedly made it all work was a trade secret—a claim frequently made about "one therapeutic system" cure-alls. After the *Wall Street Journal* began exposing Theranos with the help of disillusioned former employees of the company, Theranos accused the newspaper and the former employees of engaging in a conspiracy of lies. By the time that Theranos collapsed and Holmes was convicted of fraud, the company had squandered hundreds of millions of dollars from investors.[12]

Theranos is hardly an isolated example. According to journalist Matthew Hongoltz-Hetling, mainstream medicine now confronts an "increasingly sophisticated network of quacks" representing "America's surging medical-freedom movement." They promote what Hongoltz-Hetling calls "One True Cures," and they insist that citizens have the right to pick their own preferred health remedies and stand up to "a mystically powerful Big Pharma." The people who turn to quack remedies to try to cure their ills are sometimes condemned for being gullible. As another observer notes, however, "education is not a vaccine against folly." Individuals who pride themselves on their erudition and savvy can fall prey to medical fraud just the same as anyone else.[13]

Organized medicine's historical failures in dealing with cancer have made people especially vulnerable to quackery, given the anxiety that cancer generates. "Until the problems of cancer causation and control are fully solved, the ignorance and fear of this disease make cowards of even strong and informed people," Morris Fishbein wrote in 1965. More recent studies of cancer have borne such titles as *The Dread Disease*, or, in the case of oncologist Siddhartha Mukherjee's prizewinning book, *The Emperor of All Maladies*. Mukherjee relates appalling historical episodes: for instance, surgeons' refusal to stop performing unnecessary radical mastectomies, and South African doctor Werner Bezwoda's fraudulent research extolling megadose chemotherapy. To be sure, Mukherjee also celebrates cancer research's achievements, and cancer mortality rates have been steadily declining, thanks to improved prevention, diagnosis, and treatment. But many people still mistakenly view a cancer diagnosis as a death sentence, and effective treatments can be extremely expensive, especially for people without adequate health insurance. In addition, the shortage of proven alternatives to the standard surgery-chemotherapy-radiation regimen (sometimes referred to bitterly as "slash-poison-burn") remains a source of consternation. "It is an embarrassment. Equally embarrassing is the arrogant denial of that embarrassment," writes oncologist Azra Raza.[14]

As a result, what Susan Sontag first argued in the 1970s—that cancer represents a potent "metaphor for what is feared or deplored"—still holds true. Sontag also said that similar metaphors attach themselves to other medical conditions surrounded in mystery, as was true of AIDS when it first emerged and as later was true of COVID when it first emerged. In Sontag's words, "any important disease whose causality is murky, and for which treatment is ineffectual, tends to be awash in significance."[15] If diseases are laden with significance, so too are remedies for diseases, whether they come from inside mainstream medicine or outside it. "In the face of a scary disease, the *desire* for a ready-made solution is incredibly high," one doctor writes, and that desire can give even unproven remedies significant symbolic and political power.[16] George Stoddard, the coauthor of the anti-Krebiozen limerick that opens this book, composed another bit of doggerel mocking backers of the drug: "Want 'Krebiozen'? You fool! / It's only a word in a tiny ampoule."[17] But that one word signified very different things to opponents and proponents of Krebiozen. To the drug's opponents, it represented quackery and all that was antithetical to the principles of science. To the drug's proponents, it represented hope and freedom of choice, not to mention a powerful cudgel to wield against the likes of George Stoddard.

Battles over science and medicine have thus always been intensely personal, pointing to enduring divides over values and beliefs. Sociologists Harry Collins and Trevor Pinch have argued that medicine is "not one thing but two: medicine is a science, like other sciences, but it is also a source of succor—a source of relief or assistance in times of distress. The two faces of medicine often conflict." Medicine as science tends to privilege collective, long-term interests with the idea that trusting science over time will best serve the common good; medicine as succor tends to privilege individual, short-term interests with the idea that people should be able to use the remedies that they think will help them and shun those remedies that they think will harm them.[18]

The same conflict extends to quackery, which, according to James Harvey Young, has been viewed "from two major vantage points, one from above, the other from below." The view from above has come from the "educated, the professionally trained, the specialized in-groups like physicians, pharmacists, and bureaucratic experts." A 1969 essay by the eminent surgeon Francis Moore encapsulated this perspective. He asserted that the Krebiozen affair stemmed from an unacceptable "breach in scientific method" that produced an unjustified groundswell of support for the drug. "To the outside world, and particularly to that segment of our society that is anti-rational, anti-intellectual, and anti-scientific, the conventional trappings of science appear to be but an expression of the establishment," argued Moore. "Individuals—often unknown to science—who are fighting against the establishment become heroes to those same persons who would restrict the activity of the universities [and] do away with professors and a free press."[19]

The antiestablishment viewpoint is what Young described as the view from below, which has shunned the "quackery" label in favor of seeing nonmainstream medicine as "a component in the common man's commonsense approach to health." One historian notes that many individuals whom science branded as quacks preferred to call themselves "reformers" and "revolutionaries." They also claimed that the real quacks were representatives of organized medicine who prescribed ineffective medicines and procedures.[20] Similarly, a study of Laetrile in the 1970s observed that the drug's supporters rejected an "ideology of expertise," and instead embraced a populist ideology that insisted that people with cancer were free to select their own forms of treatment.[21] Many people over the years have shared the belief that, as another scholar describes it, organized medicine is "not only too costly, inaccessible, and ineffective but also fundamentally wrong in its most basic assumptions about the nature of illness and healing."[22]

Skepticism toward mainstream medicine persists today, some of it justified. Medical professor and author Paul Offit has noted instances in which mainstream doctors "ignore thoughtful, carefully performed studies published in excellent journals and order tests or prescribe drugs or perform cancer screenings that have clearly been shown to do more harm than good." He urges individuals to "ask good questions" of their doctors and be their own best advocates for their health.[23] Meanwhile, mainstream doctors have begun to see potential value in certain therapies advocated by individuals from outside mainstream medicine. People with cancer may be able to cope with pain, anxiety, and nausea through such mind-body techniques as autogenic training, guided imagery, mindfulness, and progressive muscle relaxation, as well as through such herbal remedies as ginger.[24] Scientists also have recognized the power of the placebo response, which some studies say may help manage cancer symptoms.[25]

The problem, according to Offit, is when people "offer placebos instead of lifesaving medicines or charge an exorbitant price for their remedies or promote therapies as harmless when they're not or encourage magical thinking and scientific denialism at a time when we can least afford it."[26] Such behavior is often driven by the conspiracy-mindedness common in quackery, and it is destructive. In one example, Ty Bollinger's "Truth about Cancer" and "Truth about Vaccines" videos have promoted unproven or disproven remedies while at the same time circulating conspiracy theories attacking mainstream medicine. Bollinger also pushed discredited theories on the 2020 US presidential election, and he helped organize demonstrations in Washington, DC, that degenerated into a violent assault on the US Capitol in January 2021.[27] Even when it is not violent, resistance to such public health measures as vaccine mandates is frequently linked to a strong mistrust of scientific authority and perceived government overreach.[28]

Ideally, colleges and universities serve as bulwarks against scientific denialism while working to promote the public welfare. The University of Illinois, for instance, developed a saliva-based rapid COVID test that the U of I then shared with other public and private institutions. Still, universities have long been inextricably intertwined with the broader business and political environment, with mixed consequences. The U of I managed not only to generate goodwill and good publicity through its COVID test; it also generated a good deal of revenue by creating a for-profit company to license the test.[29] Other times in its history, however, the U of I—like many other colleges and universities—has fallen afoul of lawmakers, donors, and other individuals outside the university over such matters as admissions procedures and controversial faculty utterances.[30] The current political climate has made matters worse for US higher education, as mistrust and resentment toward science and government have extended to public universities with increasing attacks on their autonomy.[31]

The FDA also finds itself a target. It is lambasted on one side by critics who say that the agency is overstepping its bounds and on the other side by critics who say that the agency in many ways is failing to protect the public. For example, a past president of the American Cancer Society has charged that the FDA "is now regulating research and the practice of oncology—something it was never meant to do and is not capable of doing."[32] At the same time, the agency also has been accused of being too cozy with the pharmaceutical industry and too lax toward experimental therapies for such conditions as Alzheimer's disease and amyotrophic lateral sclerosis

(ALS), even though convincing evidence showing those therapies' efficacy may be lacking. Former FDA official Joshua Sharfstein has lamented that "the growing threats to the FDA are happening at a time when the agency's expertise is especially needed."[33]

Journalism is confronting its own political and financial pressures that can make it harder to expose quackery and misinformation.[34] Credulous news stories fawn over purported medical breakthroughs, such as Theranos's claims of revolutionizing blood testing, without subjecting them to careful scrutiny. Seth Mnookin has argued that "a content-starved, cash-poor journalistic culture that gravitates toward neat narratives at the expense of messy truths" has dovetailed with online misinformation in producing "a world in which individualized notions of reality, no matter how bizarre or irrational, are repeatedly validated." Perhaps it should be no surprise that one survey has indicated that nearly 40 percent of Americans believe that unproven or disproven remedies can cure cancer.[35]

It is tempting to believe that things were much better in the past. The years just after World War II were the culmination of what has been called a "golden age" for US medicine, with doctors enjoying "social esteem and prestige along with an admiration for their work that was unprecedented in any age."[36] American higher education also was entering what is often remembered as a halcyon era marked by "the 'three P's' of prosperity, prestige, and popularity," with booming student enrollments and a vast increase in federal largesse for research in science and medicine (in contrast to today's US higher education, which is said to confront a crisis of declining enrollments and diminishing public confidence).[37] American journalism, according to communication scholar Daniel Hallin, was in its "high modern" phase, "rooted in the conviction that the primary function of the press was to serve society by providing citizens with accurate, 'unbiased' information about public affairs."[38] The FDA by the early 1960s had garnered acclaim stemming from FDA reviewer Frances Oldham Kelsey's key role in keeping thalidomide—a morning-sickness drug linked to serious birth defects—off the US market.[39]

Yet a closer look at the era reveals travails not so different from those of today. There were deep concerns over the high cost of health care alongside fears of "socialized medicine."[40] Higher education's increasing prosperity was accompanied by increasing external political pressures, including charges that it was "overrun with communists, undermined by them, infected by them."[41] McCarthyism also targeted US newsrooms, even as Senator Joseph McCarthy exploited so-called journalistic objectivity by frequently getting his red-baiting charges published without serious questioning by the press.[42] And the efforts of the FDA and other agencies to squelch health misinformation and quackery were confounded by people's endur-ing faith in what James Harvey Young described as "the countless glittering but impossible promises urged upon them by quackdom's host of clever schemers."[43]

This was the era that gave rise to Krebiozen, and the story of its rise and fall is as relevant as ever, for it provides important historical context in understanding the turbulence that currently buffets medicine and other professions and institutions. The Krebiozen saga shows that charges of conspiracy, elitism, and un-Americanism directed against the educational, scientific, and medical establishment are nothing new; neither is uncritical news coverage of what turns out to be quackery. And Krebiozen was in fact quackery: it displayed all the characteristics that Young identified as being typical of medical fraud.

Krebiozen's sponsors exploited the fear of painful surgery and radia-tion to promote a nontoxic wonder remedy that the drug's backers main-tained was the scientific key to treating cancer. Krebiozen's "one cause, one therapeutic system" theory postulated that all living cells possessed a growth regulator that could be isolated from horse serum and used to fight malignant tumors in humans. The medicine's sponsors insisted that the full details of the drug's composition and production were a business secret. Proponents of the drug frequently compared Andrew Ivy to Louis Pasteur and other visionaries whose scientific breakthroughs were initially scorned by mainstream medicine. Krebiozen's backers also charged that the AMA had conspired to crush the drug, charges similar to those previ-ously leveled by such cancer quacks as Norman Baker and Harry Hoxsey. Evidence suggested that after Stevan Durovic was unable to win support for a hypertension medicine that he called "Kositerin," he rebranded the exact same concoction as a cancer medicine called "Krebiozen"—a rebranding to adjust to circumstances. The medicine was advertised via such means as a pulp magazine trumpeting the miraculous results that cancer patients had experienced: "DOOMED TO DIE—THEY STILL LIVE!" The drug's support-ers declared that they stood for health-care freedom, continually vexing the AMA, the FDA, and the National Cancer Institute (NCI). In time, according to bank records introduced at the fraud trial, Krebiozen became a multi-million-dollar enterprise.[44]

The Krebiozen story was not bereft of good intentions or good ideas. Before his involvement with the drug, Andrew Ivy was the last person whom anyone would have compared with the likes of Baker or Hoxsey. Instead, he was much more like Linus Pauling, the later proponent of vitamin C as a cancer therapy. Ivy was widely acknowledged as a distinguished scien-tist with impeccable academic credentials. Few people suggested that he promoted Krebiozen just to get rich, in contrast with Stevan Durovic, who would be accused by the US government of extracting a vast sum of money out of the country and depositing it into overseas accounts. Ivy always would insist that he wanted only to get an impartial test of the hypothesis that he said he had developed out of the existing scientific literature: that people carried within them a natural cancer inhibitor, most likely a hormone produced by the reticuloendothelial system. (Krebiozen's supporters said that cancer patients needed the drug to manage their conditions just as diabetics needed insulin to manage glucose levels.) Subsequent cancer research has suggested that in some ways, at least, Ivy was on the right track. Scientists have discovered the existence of tumor-suppressor genes. Studies have linked insulin and other hormones to the metabolism of cancer. And one of the most promising new areas of research and treatment—immunotherapy—harnesses the body's natural defenses against cancer.[45]

What is more, Krebiozen users were not all hapless dupes. Many of them had felt abandoned by mainstream medicine or, as in the case of Rachel Carson, had been misled by their doctors about the gravity of their conditions. For them, Krebiozen seemed a rational choice. "I'm not expecting miracles," said Carson of Krebiozen. "As far as I've been able to learn it will do no harm, so what do I have to lose?"[46] If people subsequently decided that the drug did not work for them (as turned out to be the case with Carson), they simply could stop taking it. Other cancer patients and their loved ones were convinced that Krebiozen was the one thing keeping them alive.

In the end, though, Krebiozen turned out to be a hoax, regardless of whether it was planned as such. The medicine always would remain a secret remedy that was never scientifically shown to be effective. Stevan Durovic blocked efforts by federal agencies to witness the drug's manufacture from start to finish. Patient records intended to demonstrate Krebiozen's efficacy never met the standards set by the NCI to justify a clinical test of the drug. Eventually, Durovic and Ivy would alienate some of their most steadfast allies after they repeatedly failed to uphold their promises for Krebiozen. Still, the hoax persisted for years because so many people wanted so fervently to believe that the drug worked. Why that passionate belief endured for as long as it did is a key question that this book seeks to answer.

Chapter 1, "Substance X," examines the environment that fostered the Krebiozen controversy. The post–World War II era in US higher education was filled with promise and excitement, as veterans using GI Bill benefits flocked to college campuses. The University of Illinois had installed a progressive new president, George Stoddard. His administration oversaw the creation of innovative programs and the hiring of scores of faculty members and administrators. One of the most prominent new hires was Andrew Ivy, picked to lead the U of I's medical programs in Chicago. But not everyone was happy about the rapid changes at the state university. Some academic units erupted in open revolt, while conservative critics off campus charged that the U of I was promoting unpatriotic and antireligious thought. For his part, Ivy was preoccupied with a mysterious new medicine that had been introduced to him by a stranger visiting from Argentina. The medicine was called "Substance X," and Stevan Durovic would not tell Ivy how it was made, but he did say that it could treat cancer. After determining that the substance was not toxic, Ivy tested it on human patients. Their responses—and Ivy's concerns that Durovic and his brother might leave the country and take the new drug with them—persuaded Ivy to announce the medicine (rechristened "Krebiozen") to the world.

Chapter 2, "Krebiozen Does Not Exist," discusses the fallout from Ivy's 1951 announcement. It generated headlines across the country and prompted desperate pleas for the drug from as far away as Brazil. The American Medical Association was unimpressed and began investigating Krebiozen, even as some of Ivy's closest colleagues frantically tried to steer him clear of the drug and the Durovic brothers. After an AMA report found no validity to Ivy's claims for the medicine, Ivy blasted the report as biased and unscientific, and he won sympathy from individuals who disliked the AMA for its monopolistic practices and its hostility toward public health insurance. Although at first the U of I had publicly expressed support for Ivy, President Stoddard feared that the controversy was damaging the university's reputation and morale. He asked two faculty committees to study Krebiozen. When the committees could not uncover convincing evidence of the drug's efficacy or obtain full cooperation from the Durovics, Stoddard issued his own verdict in late 1952: Krebiozen was a fake.

Chapter 3, "Conspiracies and Circuses," describes the vehement reaction of Ivy's allies to Stoddard's pronouncement. Those allies included lawmakers from Chicago's West Side, where the U of I's medical programs were located. The lawmakers saw the programs as a valuable source of patronage by giving preference to politically connected applicants for jobs in the U of I hospital and enrollment in the U of I medical school. Other state legislators simply did not like Stoddard. After Ivy charged that the AMA had conspired with two Chicago-area businesspeople to kill Krebiozen, the state legislature launched hearings, partly to bolster Ivy and embarrass Stoddard. Those hearings would last for several months and turn into a public circus. Amid the hearings, the U of I Board of Trustees voted no confidence in Stoddard and his chief lieutenant, Provost Coleman Griffith. The vote had been called by former U of I football great Red Grange, who had been elected to the board on an anticommunist Republican slate. Stoddard and Griffith promptly resigned, and Stoddard blamed it all on Krebiozen, triggering outrage over political interference at the university. In early 1954, the legislative hearings fizzled to a close, with no conspiracy having been uncovered.

Chapter 4, "A Fair Test," relates how Krebiozen became a nationwide cause. Writer Herbert Bailey published a fiercely polemical book in 1955 that trumpeted Krebiozen's miraculous benefits and attacked Krebiozen's opponents, including Stoddard and the alleged conspirators against the drug. When at the same time Stoddard published his own book questioning the drug's existence, Ivy at first sought to have Stoddard's book suppressed and then sued Stoddard for libel. The controversy stirred by the rival books captured the attention of people who saw Ivy as a persecuted maverick. Columnist Drew Pearson wrote sympathetic articles about Krebiozen, and film star Gloria Swanson touted the drug on television and spoke at fund-raising dinners for Ivy. Organizations called the Citizens Emergency Committee for Krebiozen and the Ivy Cancer Leagues drew support from across the country. Members of Congress, particularly Illinois Senator Paul Douglas, urged organized medicine to give Krebiozen an unbiased test that, if successful, would allow licensing and commercial sale of the drug. (Krebiozen was being distributed for investigational use in exchange for a nine-dollar-fifty-cent donation per ampule.) In 1961, a federal judge asked the US Department of Health, Education, and Welfare to conduct such a test, making it seem as though a resolution to the Krebiozen controversy finally was at hand.

Chapter 5, "Nothing but Creatine," explains why that test never happened. Ivy and Stevan Durovic did not comply with the National Cancer Institute's ground rules for evaluating new therapies. In 1962, after the thalidomide tragedy, Congress granted the Food and Drug Administration authority to ensure the efficacy of new drugs. The FDA subsequently began an investigation of Krebiozen, with inspectors visiting Durovic's laboratory in Chicago and rifling through the trash of Krebiozen proponents. Claiming government harassment, Durovic withdrew his application to the FDA for continuing experimental use of the drug. The medicine already was being taken by people ranging from Freda DeKnight of *Ebony* magazine to Rachel Carson, the author of *Silent Spring*. With the US government now banning interstate shipment of Krebiozen, panicked users of the drug picketed the White House and demanded that the government continue to allow access to the medicine. In September 1963, an FDA team led by pioneering African American scientist Alma LeVant Hayden reported that its tests of Krebiozen had shown it to be creatine, a common amino acid derivative that was of no use against cancer. Soon afterward, the NCI said that its review of patient case histories indicated that no government test of Krebiozen was warranted.

Chapter 6, "The Emperor's New Clothes," describes how Senator Douglas claimed that the government was deliberately smearing Krebiozen. He tried to arrange an independent test of the drug through the intercession of President Lyndon B. Johnson, who had just taken office; that attempt fell through after Ivy and Durovic again did not cooperate fully. In 1964, Ivy and the Durovic brothers were indicted on fraud charges. The subsequent trial in Chicago would last nine months and be overseen by the famously irascible Judge Julius Hoffman (who later would garner added notoriety for his handling of the "Chicago Seven" trial of antiwar activists). The prosecution quoted from Hans Christian Andersen's tale of the vain emperor who is swindled by two strangers pretending to weave a set of magic garments; according to the prosecution, the emperor in this case was Ivy, the swindlers were the Durovics, and the new clothes were Krebiozen. The defense cited "The Walrus and the Carpenter" in suggesting that Krebiozen had been gobbled up by the predatory AMA, like the oysters gobbled up by the walrus and carpenter in the Lewis Carroll poem. After fraught deliberations, the jury acquitted the defendants on all charges. (One juror was later convicted on tampering charges and imprisoned.) Krebiozen supporters tried one last time to win interstate shipment of the drug, staging a sit-in at FDA headquarters until police carried them away. It was to no avail: Stevan Durovic left the country after being indicted for tax evasion, and interest in Krebiozen dwindled until Illinois, the only state where the drug could legally be obtained, quietly banned the medicine in 1973.

The conclusion—"What Ever Happened to Doctor Ivy?"—takes its title from a 1964 critical profile of Andrew Ivy in *Life* magazine. The conclusion reviews the history of the Krebiozen case and ponders why Ivy and the other principals in the Krebiozen case acted the way that they did.

• • •

Unproven remedies can give hope to sufferers of medical maladies, but mainstream science and medicine offer their own causes for optimism. "We have a right to hope that cancer [will someday] fall within the range of the understandable and the curable," said George Stoddard in 1955. "It will take time. It will take the kind of research that is being carried on patiently and undramatically in hundreds of laboratories over the world." Stoddard contrasted the hopes that he saw as being wisely invested in medical science with the "false hopes" that he saw as being unwisely invested in the likes of Krebiozen. James Harvey Young similarly lamented the damage that quackery wreaks. "Quackery, like poverty, bigotry, and violence, must now be seen as a primary and stubborn challenge to our intelligence and will," he wrote, adding that "paradoxically, such a perspective may offer greater hope than the more naively hopeful view" that quackery might one day fade away.[47]

Andrew Ivy saw things differently. "Some have said, 'We should not give false hope.' This is sophistry," he commented late in his career when he was largely limited to treating dying cancer patients at no charge with what was widely viewed as a discredited remedy. Ivy believed that sometimes hope was all that doctors could provide, as opposed to charging enormous sums for standard therapies that did not help in terminal cases. Another doctor reported just such a case involving a man dying of cancer who begged to be given Krebiozen. After the doctor reluctantly obliged his wishes, the man's condition rapidly and dramatically improved, his tumors having "melted like snow balls on a hot stove." The doctor believed that the patient was thriving purely from the placebo response, which he confirmed when he injected the man with nothing but water while claiming it still to be Krebiozen and saw the patient's remarkable response continue. When the man heard independently of his doctor that the AMA had found Krebiozen to be worthless, however, he swiftly declined and died, having lost his only source of hope.[48]

What follows, then, is more than a book about cancer and quackery. It also is a book that ponders what people place their hope in and how they struggle to maintain that hope when they face their gravest challenges, health-wise and otherwise.

CHAPTER 1

Substance X

To understand how Krebiozen sparked so much controversy over so many years, one first needs to know something of the time and place from which the drug emerged. Krebiozen was born in the wake of World War II and at the beginning of the atomic age and the Cold War, a period that brought about vast and sometimes unsettling changes. Few institutions were affected as profoundly by those changes—and by Krebiozen itself—as the University of Illinois (U of I).

Like other colleges and universities, the U of I had struggled during the 1930s and the early 1940s. The Depression compelled the university to cut faculty salaries while forcing many students to reduce their food budgets to just a few cents per day. Then the war came, and enrollment plummeted as a large number of students joined the military. In addition, an external review by the American Council on Education in 1943 criticized the U of I's "conservative and sometimes reactionary senior professors and administrators," who made the university "not a desirable place at which to work."[1]

In the spring of 1945 the U of I Board of Trustees approached George Stoddard to become the new university president, replacing Arthur Willard, who was about to reach mandatory retirement age. Stoddard had served as director of the Iowa Child Welfare Research Station and as University of Iowa graduate dean before becoming New York state commissioner of education. He was in only his third year in New York and was reluctant to take another job so soon, but he and his family were eager to return to the lifestyle that a midwestern state university afforded. Moreover, as Stoddard later remembered, "Illinois itself was at the heart center of the Middle West—a leader in population, agriculture, industry, transportation, and

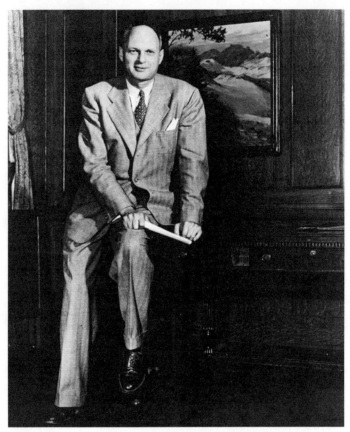

George Stoddard officially became University of Illinois president in 1946. He would oversee vast and rapid change at the university. (Courtesy of the University of Illinois at Urbana-Champaign Archives, image 0007804)

financial power. In the near future I was to hear the president of a sister state university refer to the University of Illinois as 'a sleeping giant.'"[2] At the age of forty-seven when he accepted his new position, Stoddard was nearly twenty years younger than Willard, and he became one of the youngest presidents in U of I history. The Champaign-Urbana *Courier* hailed his hiring by saying that "good feeling today is unanimous" on campus.[3]

That good feeling continued after the war ended. The *Daily Illini* student newspaper reserved a full page in its first issue of 1946 to herald the promise of a new year "when education for peace takes the place of schooling for destruction, a bright and busy year of building back, a year when hatreds shall fade in the dawning hope of brotherhood."[4] Congress had enacted the Serviceman's Readjustment Act of 1944—popularly known as the GI

Bill—to ease veterans' reassimilation into civilian life, with education benefits included in the legislation. Few people foresaw just how many veterans would take advantage. By the fall of 1946 more than a million of them had descended on college campuses across the country, and enrollment would continue to expand through the rest of the decade.[5]

The U of I experienced abrupt, unprecedented demand as it became the second-largest university in the country. The student population at the Champaign-Urbana campus in central Illinois topped 19,000 in 1947, up 60 percent from just two years before; veteran enrollment alone surpassed 11,000 at its peak. More than three thousand veteran students were married with nearly one thousand children.[6] The university quickly opened satellite campuses at Chicago's Navy Pier and in the Illinois city of Galesburg to help handle the crunch. In Champaign-Urbana, people were housed in the university's ice rink and football stadium, and barracks-like accommodations were installed on the drill field and parade grounds. The veterans proved to be excellent students, many of whom reveled in the campus atmosphere. "I actually had a hell of a good time going to school," one veteran recalled of his return to the U of I after three years in the military.[7]

The new energy was palpable, shaking up not only the university, but also the surrounding community. Champaign-Urbana residents were urged to open their homes and offer room and board to the surge of students. Those students fortunate enough to find accommodations on campus created governing councils, intramural sports teams, and newspapers to serve university housing units. A group of returning veterans in wheelchairs helped establish a groundbreaking program to accommodate disabilities. Thanks to those students' efforts, the U of I became a global leader in accessible building design.[8] Other students displayed heightened social consciousness by fighting segregation in local restaurants, theaters, and swimming pools. They could do only so much to improve the lot of African Americans, who then constituted less than 1 percent of the student body. Even so, many Black students—some of whom were returning veterans themselves—joined the battle against discrimination while holding their own in the classroom.[9]

During the war, women on campus had taken over leadership roles previously reserved for men. Now, though, they increasingly found themselves "knee deep in diapers and dirty dishes," as one historian has put it. That did not mean that they meekly reassumed subservient status. After President Stoddard proposed a new women's curriculum stressing home economics, a female reporter wrote in the *Courier* newspaper that she did "not approve of the new curriculum even if it helps women 'adjust to the world in which they are to live,' any more than I would approve of courses designed to enable members of the Negro or Jewish minorities [to] 'adjust' to the difficult situations in which they sometimes regrettably find themselves." However, the university did hire a new dean of women named Miriam Shelden, who had served as a reserve commander in the US Navy. Shelden became a vigorous advocate for female students and for students of color.[10]

Shelden was in her midthirties when she joined the U of I, in keeping with the emphasis on new, younger leadership established by the hiring of President Stoddard himself; several other new deans also were in their thirties and forties. Stoddard later said that, for a brief time at least, the U of I Board of Trustees and the state legislature seemed determined to do whatever it took to build a world-class institution. The president was able to procure an across-the-board 24 percent average increase in faculty salaries. New commerce dean Howard Bowen recalled hearing that "the University of Illinois had more operating funds than any university in the previous history of the world. I never checked the validity of this statement, but I can attest that the university was exceptionally affluent during the late 1940s."[11]

Under Stoddard, the U of I developed its Institute of Labor and Industrial Relations, Institute of Communications Research, and Institute of Government and Public Affairs to accompany the Institute of Aviation that had opened in 1945 along with the world's largest university airport. The university also turned a onetime rural estate into a conference center called Allerton Park. In July 1949, the new center hosted a conference that had far-reaching effects. The National Association of Educational Broadcasters subsequently moved its headquarters to the U of I, and that organization eventually helped lay the groundwork for the Public Broadcasting Service and National Public Radio.[12]

Stoddard said that the most important achievement during his presidency was the inauguration of the Festival of Contemporary Arts in 1948. The annual festivals drew large crowds to the university to be bemused by the latest in nonrepresentational art. When asked to explain one such artwork, a festival juror was apologetic: "I don't understand the painting myself!" Music, theater, and literature were pondered and celebrated as well. Among the many luminaries whom the festivals brought to campus were director Harold Clurman; composers Aaron Copland and Igor Stravinsky; and writers Dylan Thomas, Archibald MacLeish, Randall Jarrell, and Howard Mumford Jones, the last of whom called on young people to "revolt and again demoralize the dead weight of conformity that now lies upon us."[13]

The sciences—already a U of I strength—were not neglected. The university built the world's largest betatron particle accelerator for research and placed another betatron at its medical center in Chicago to treat cancer.

By assembling the ILLIAC I digital computer, the U of I became a leader in computer science; at the same time, it became a leader in solid-state physics. Before the war, the physics department had found it difficult to attract star faculty to central Illinois ("I love subways and I hate cows," one professor in New York had said). That situation now changed, thanks to more money and a collegial department that did not discriminate against Jews or the progressively minded. John Bardeen, who recently had coinvented the transistor at Bell Labs, joined the Illinois faculty in 1951, and he subsequently became the only two-time awardee of the Nobel Prize in Physics.[14]

Of all the high-profile new hires at the U of I, though, the most impressive at the time may have been that of Andrew Conway Ivy. One of the world's preeminent physiologists, Ivy had trained at the University of Chicago under the legendary Anton J. "Ajax" Carlson, known for his hectoring query aimed at students and fellow scientists in a thick Swedish accent: "Vot iss de effidence?" Ivy embodied a similar critical exactitude at Northwestern University, where he headed the physiology and pharmacology division for more than twenty years. When an Italian doctor asserted in 1934 that the human being was a "television machine" capable of transmitting and receiving extrasensory images, Ivy was politely but pronouncedly skeptical: "Such reports have come in from time to time during the last 10 years. The difficulty is that when studied in critical detail and with knowledge of modern physical and chemical achievement, these reports are subject to doubt."[15]

Ivy also emulated his mentor Carlson in tackling a vast array of research topics. They included the fight against alcohol and drug addiction, the search for effective treatments for polio and syphilis, the deleterious effects of prolonged work hours and of vitamin deficiencies, the safe conversion of seawater into drinking water, and the physiological impact of parachute jumping. Ivy conducted some of that work while serving as scientific director of the US Naval Medical Research Institute during the war. He was especially renowned for his research on peptic ulcers and gastroenterology, and he claimed to have "discovered and helped establish the existence of more hormones than any man alive." Ivy collaborated on more than fifteen hundred scientific papers and trained more than five thousand medical students. His reputation grew to the point that when Anton Carlson was asked what his own greatest contribution to physiology had been, he replied simply, "Dr. Ivy."[16]

In 1946, when Ivy was fifty-three years old, the U of I lured him from Northwestern by creating an entirely new position for him: vice president in charge of the U of I's Chicago professional colleges, consisting of the

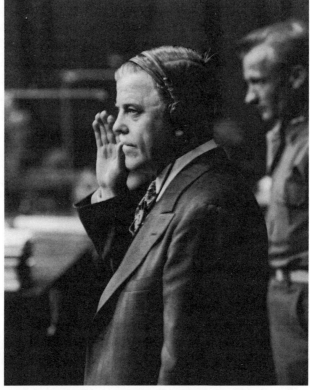

Andrew Ivy testifying as an expert witness at the Nuremberg Trials in December 1946. *Time* magazine at that time called him "the conscience of U.S. science." (Wikimedia Commons)

College of Medicine, the College of Dentistry, and the College of Pharmacy. Ivy's new job coincided with the American Medical Association nominating him to be an expert adviser to the Nuremberg war crimes tribunal. He testified for the prosecution in the trial of Nazi doctors who were charged with committing atrocities during spurious medical experiments on prisoners. Ivy helped write the Nuremberg Code of medical ethics, which asserted that "voluntary consent of the human subject is absolutely essential." Not long afterward, he also collaborated on a pamphlet for the Anti-Defamation League of B'nai B'rith denouncing racial and religious bias in American universities. "Discrimination in education is a national scandal," the pamphlet proclaimed. "Its evils should be obvious to all." It was in response to such activities and declarations of principle that *Time* magazine called Ivy "the conscience of U.S. science."[17]

Ivy was more complicated than media coverage made him seem. During cross-examination of Ivy in the Nuremberg trial, the defense had asked him about medical research performed on prisoners in his home state of Illinois. He replied that he chaired a committee appointed by the Illinois governor to study the issue, and the committee had found the prisoner research to be wholly ethical. Although the committee did exist, it had yet to meet; Ivy had produced its "findings" by himself for the sake of the trial, an action that verged on perjury. While he was at Northwestern, Ivy also had tangled with animal welfare activists who objected to his using dogs from the Chicago city pound for experiments. The activists sued him along with Northwestern's president and medical dean. One woman testified that she had visited Ivy's lab and found dogs in cages "about as big as my hat boxes." The woman added that when she tried to rescue one dog, Ivy chased after her, "sank his claws in the dog's neck, and flung" the animal on the ground before hauling it back to the lab.[18]

Such incidents did little to blemish Ivy's public image. The courts dismissed the cruelty charges against him and the other Northwestern officials, and Ivy stoutly defended the use of animals in medical research. "We'd get discouraged if it were not for the other letters and reports we receive showing that our work has saved human lives," he told a reporter. "We often wonder how much our critics have done to help sick soldiers or sick children." Ivy proved adept at cultivating the press. *Time* wrote that he was "as American as baseball." One 1947 newspaper profile acknowledged that he did have his faults—he wore loud ties, and he drove too fast. Even then, said the newspaper, "the police agree he drives skillfully and safely."[19] The new U of I vice president also was skillful in obtaining funds to expand the university's medical facilities. Along with installing the betatron for cancer therapy, the Chicago professional colleges opened a new Aeromedical and Physical Environment Laboratory and began building a hospital addition, increasing external grants more than fivefold between 1946 and 1950.[20]

In short, the University of Illinois seemed to be flourishing right after the war. President Stoddard would fondly recall those years as representing "not only the 'salad days' for Illinois but also for the whole structure of higher education in the United States."[21]

• • •

Salad days are often not quite so "salad" as later remembered, and such was the case with the U of I. The speedy, progressive change at a previously staid and conservative institution sparked a backlash against Stoddard's leadership—a backlash that reflected seismic changes in US higher education.

According to historian John R. Thelin, the early twentieth century had given rise to a group of university presidents who, through savvy public relations, came to be seen as "heroic" and as "visionary pioneers." The U of I had been led by just such a heroic president, Edmund J. James, from 1904 to 1920. He was credited with transforming the university and giving it a global reputation. "James dreamed big dreams and had a special talent for promotion and publicity," a biographer has written. James successfully pushed for larger state appropriations to support his ambitions for the U of I, and his influence became such that "no Illinois politician dared be openly hostile to the university."[22]

Stoddard would have no such luck. The era after World War II would see the rise of what Clark Kerr described as the "multiversity," with the typical university changing from a unified, insular community into a far more complex entity representing "so many things to so many different people that it must, of necessity, be partially at war with itself." A university president's ideal function shifted from being a charismatic visionary into being what Kerr called a "mediator" who had to answer to multiple publics (alumni, donors, politicians, and so forth) holding competing interests that ranged from "quite legitimate" to "quite frivolous." The president-as-mediator had to balance two conflicting roles: keeping the peace and pushing for progress. As a peacekeeper, said Kerr, the president was obligated to maintain productive relationships not only among students, faculty, staff, and trustees but also "between the internal environment of the academic community and the external society that surrounds and sometimes almost engulfs it." As an agent of progress, the president was obligated to prod the university forward in the face of resistance to change, responding proactively to the knowledge explosion and population explosion that characterized the postwar years.[23]

Stoddard readily embraced the agent-of-progress role as U of I president, but he seemed less amenable to the peacekeeper role, particularly in trying to appease what he viewed as frivolous or foolish interests. By his own admission, he sometimes was "guilty of the cold eye and dour look,"[24] and he was not shy about expressing his views on controversial subjects. Thus he would stir anger among some constituencies in Illinois even before he was formally installed as president.

Stoddard had been raised in a churchgoing Methodist family in Pennsylvania coal country, but at a young age he adopted decidedly liberal views toward organized religion, eventually gravitating toward Unitarianism. While leading the Iowa Child Welfare Research Station, he also became a passionate proponent of the idea that children's intelligence was shaped at least as much by environment as it was by heredity. He outlined his perspective in his 1943 book *The Meaning of Intelligence*, saying that the truly feebleminded were individuals who had been "systematically drugged with the vapors of dogma, superstition, and pseudo logic." If anyone missed the point, Stoddard went on to write that "man-made concepts, such as *devils, witches, totems, taboos, hell-fire, original sin, divine right, predestination, reincarnation, salvation-through-death-in-battle*, and *divine revelation*" had "distorted the intellectual processes of millions of persons over the centuries."[25]

Stoddard's book was directed toward an academic audience, but it came to the attention of Bishop James A. Griffin of the Roman Catholic diocese in Springfield, Illinois. Bishop Griffin was known for his attacks on Hollywood pictures that he believed to be immoral, having once charged that film canisters contained "thousands of feet of movie film, coiled like serpents, ready to pour their venom into the souls of our children." After Stoddard's hiring at the U of I was announced, Griffin took to the pulpit in September 1945 to attack the president-elect: "As long as men like George Dinsmore Stoddard sound the keynote of modern education, our 'last chance'—a return to spiritual values—will never be realized. What are you, citizens of Illinois, going to do about it?" Stoddard's pledge to respect the religious views of all students seemed to mollify the bishop, and Stoddard assumed the U of I presidency as scheduled the following year.[26]

Soon there were new concerns that initially did not involve Stoddard himself. In the war's immediate aftermath, the U of I welcomed avowedly leftist speakers and artists to campus. Mollie Lieber of the American Youth for Democracy (AYD) told her audience that the "Soviet people have as their objective the reconstruction of their country and desire only to live in peace." Paul Robeson touted the AYD as a "very progressive organization" after singing for an enthusiastic crowd of sixty-five hundred people at the university. "It is obvious nonsense that the Russians can take this country over," Robeson added. "The guys who go on a Red scare are the same who have created the Negro situation in the South and the anti-Semitism that exist[s] today."[27]

However, by the spring of 1947 when Robeson performed at the U of I, the Cold War already had taken hold and fears of Russia and communism were growing. In a front-page editorial, the *Daily Illini* denounced the AYD as a communist front. A Republican state lawmaker from Champaign, Charles Clabaugh, sponsored a bill in the Illinois legislature to target such groups. "Universities of America have been the breeding grounds of a series of insidious, communist-inspired organizations which have sought to instill in the hearts of American youth contempt and hatred for ideals to which the people of this great nation have been dedicated," the bill declared. It denied university facility access to "any subversive, seditious and un-American organization." What became known as the Clabaugh Act was signed into law in August 1947 and would remain in effect for decades.[28]

George Stoddard was a liberal who rejected red-baiting, but by no stretch of the imagination was he a radical. "There is a militant, statist, paranoiac element in communism that comes after us," he said in a speech. "Our freedom of choice is reduced to running or resisting." Under Stoddard, a new university security office was tasked with investigating what security officer Joseph Ewers described as "any statement or action termed even slightly subversive or 'pink'."[29] Suspicion fell on a number of U of I faculty, at least four of whom were forced to leave the university for alleged communist ties. As for the rest of the campus, though, Ewers told the U of I Board of Trustees that there were no more than "10 or 15 persons with 'will-o-the-wisp' subversive ideas." In one instance, when a radical faction tried to control a group called the Student-Community Interracial Committee, other members ousted the radicals by disbanding the organization altogether and then reforming it under another name.[30]

Such efforts at self-policing did not appease certain members of the state legislature. Republican Paul Broyles from Mount Vernon in southern Illinois sponsored anticommunist bills that were opposed by many U of I faculty as well as by President Stoddard; a so-called Broyles commission also investigated Illinois universities. According to one report, the commission "could not discover a single teacher in Illinois who was a Communist or advocated communism in his teaching."[31] The university's political critics were not limited to one region of the state or one political party. The American Council on Education's 1943 review of the university had been prompted by scathing charges from Illinois attorney general George Barrett, a Chicago Republican. Barrett claimed that the U of I had "been on the downgrade since 1934 when control was taken over by a board of trustees who were not the choice of the people but were hand-picked by the downstate Democratic machine and the Kelly-Nash machine" in Chicago. Noting that it had found no support for Barrett's allegations, the education council said that "the present situation is fraught with grave dangers for the future of the University. Educational issues may become confused with political or partisan considerations—if indeed this has not already occurred." Six years later in 1949, U of I medical dean John Youmans was targeted by Democratic state legislator Vito Marzullo, who was from Chicago's West Side, where the U of I medical programs were located. Marzullo and his allies charged that Youmans—who had been hired under Stoddard—had turned the medical school into a "dumping ground" for "out-of-state cronies with phony titles." Youmans soon left the U of I to go to Vanderbilt University, saying that there was "less undesirable pressure" there.[32]

The most persistent criticisms of the U of I during the Stoddard years came from Republicans in central Illinois, with the criticisms reflecting deep-seated political and cultural divisions. Democratic US senator Paul Douglas of Illinois half-jokingly blamed such divisions on natural history. Thousands of years previously, the glaciers had stopped halfway down the state, resulting in less fertile soil and less prosperity in southern Illinois; consequently, Democrats enjoyed more political support in that part of the state. In central Illinois, however, the glaciers had left some of the richest soil in the world, producing more prosperity, more conservatism, and more Republicans. Therefore—as recalled by the senator's aide Howard Shuman—Douglas would tell the "lonely Democrats" of central Illinois that it was not their fault that they were perpetually in the minority: "They were really fighting against the glaciers."[33]

Stoddard and many of the new hires who followed him to Champaign-Urbana seemed predestined to fight the same battle. The *News-Gazette*, a conservative Champaign newspaper, became a staunch opponent of the Stoddard regime. In May 1950, its managing editor wrote of a conversation that he claimed to have had with a group of his friends. "Right in our own town the University is being allowed to slip out of its traditional sound bed-rock educational program," the editor quoted one friend as saying. "We don't want a Harvard or [University of] Chicago down here in the black dirt country. Let the east and the big cities espouse those kinds of universities."[34]

Stoddard faced attacks on multiple fronts. He chaired the US National Commission for the United Nations Educational, Scientific, and Cultural Organization (UNESCO), and therefore he was deemed to be an internationalist, much like his good friend Adlai Stevenson, a Democrat who was elected Illinois governor in 1948. "Along with a lot of our readers, we think UNESCO is pretty much a waste of time," said the editorial page of the *Chicago Tribune*, whose conservative influence reached across Illinois. Stoddard said that he worked for UNESCO on his personal time as opposed to university time, which the *Tribune* said was fine as long as he did not "neglect the university for world saving." In fact, that was precisely what the *News-Gazette* accused Stoddard of doing. "The president, we regret to say, is away a great deal of the time," the paper wrote of Stoddard in 1950, suggesting that he was shirking his duties in preventing the U of I's pernicious slippage from its traditional virtues.[35]

The U of I's budget also came under fire; not everyone was pleased to hear talk of the university having more operating dollars than any other school in history. "Ever since President Stoddard has been in the driver's seat, the University has had money for practically anything it wanted to do," the *News-Gazette* editorialized. "Just as most of us would do personally if our pockets were full of money, it has spent freely and sometimes fool-ishly."[36] The days in which the Illinois legislature granted funds for big salary hikes and hiring sprees ended, followed by struggles in the state capitol in Springfield over university appropriations. At the same time, fears of left-ist influence at the U of I intensified. In 1949, two Republican lawmakers proposed cutting funding for the Institute of Labor and Industrial Rela-tions and firing certain of its faculty for allegedly "red" ideas. Among other things, the institute had sponsored a panel that argued that the Taft-Hartley antiunion law should be repealed. President Stoddard and the university successfully protected the institute's funding, but its director resigned.[37]

The concerns over the university's direction came to a head in 1950, when the U of I's College of Commerce erupted in open warfare.[38] President Stod-dard and Provost Coleman Griffith had hired Howard Bowen as commerce dean in 1947 with the mandate to reinvigorate the college, which had a repu-tation for being inbred and complacent as well as for emphasizing business training over academic research. Bowen took advantage of the university's open coffers right after the war in making fifty-five faculty appointments with a particular eye to raising the economics department's research profile. Within three years, professors at other universities were praising the U of I for having developed one of the top economics programs in the country. But such rapid and dramatic improvements came at a cost. New faculty had been brought in from the outside at higher salaries than those earned by faculty whose hirings had predated Bowen's arrival as dean; Bowen also had overruled several proposed promotions among the old guard of professors. Resentments grew. Bowen later acknowledged that he was inexperienced in academic administration and that he had tried to push certain changes too aggressively. When he shared his uneasiness with Provost Griffith and President Stoddard, however, they told him not to relent.

The result, as Bowen recalled, was "general turmoil. Committees and caucuses were organized, innumerable meetings were held, press releases were issued, debates were staged, abortive efforts at reconciliation were launched, and mountains were made out of insignificant episodes or slips of the tongue." The *News-Gazette* became the mouthpiece of anti-Bowen faculty, one of whom said privately that he "would get old Bowen thrown out for raping a heifer if I could arrange it." Charges grew in the press that the U of I had embraced what the *Chicago Tribune* called "quack econom-ics"—that is, New Deal–style Keynesian economics. When a U of I faculty committee investigating the controversy reported that "there has been no indoctrination of ideas foreign to our democratic system," the Hearst-owned *Chicago Herald-American* blared the news under the headline "Deny Reds Rule U. of I. Faculty."[39]

The commerce controversy coincided with the outbreak of the Korean War and the start of US Senator Joseph McCarthy's anticommunist witch-hunts; Russia already had announced that it had denotated an atomic bomb, and communists had recently taken over China. Cold War tensions boiled over in a raucous Illinois Republican convention in Peoria in August 1950. The party ejected Chicago business executive Chester Davis from its slate of candidates for the popularly elected U of I Board of Trustees. Davis was branded as one of the trustees who had recruited Stoddard to Illinois. The replacement on the Republican ticket was former Illinois football great Harold "Red" Grange, about whom it was said that "the only thing red about him is his hair and his blood." At the same convention, state lawmaker Ora Dillavou accused the U of I of harboring fifty "socialists, communists, or pinks" on its faculty. Stoddard's pugnacity came to the fore. He sent Dillavou a form with fifty blank spaces to be filled in with the names of the purported miscreants. Each page of the form was headed with the words, "Mr. Dillavou's List." Dillavou retorted that it was Stoddard's job to uncover subversives, while fellow Republican Charles Clabaugh told the *News-Gazette* that the "people's confidence in the administration of the University of Illinois has been shaken."[40]

To compound the university's troubles, the School of Music also became embroiled in highly publicized turmoil over its leadership, reinforcing the impression that the U of I under Stoddard was spiraling out of control. After thirty-four music professors called for a vote of no confidence in their director John Kuypers, he resigned in December 1950. Howard Bowen suffered the same fate at the same time. The faculty committee that had found no evidence of radical teachings in the College of Commerce also said that the college had fallen victim to "a failure in human relations and a failure in administration." Bowen stepped down as dean, and he soon left the U of I altogether to go on to a distinguished career as president of Grinnell College and then as president of the University of Iowa.[41]

The darkening of the mood at the U of I within such a short period was striking. At the start of 1946, the *Daily Illini* had greeted the new year with joyous confidence and hopes for world peace; now it was saying farewell to the old year of 1950 by warning that "our civilization is threatened—truly for the first time—by a ruthless, robot creed. World Communism, monstrous, powerful, militant in its growing immensity, makes all its adherents alien—animal and unreasoning, with souls blank of compassion—fearless men taught to hate and to conquer." President Stoddard, at least, seemed to have weathered the year's turbulence. The *Chicago Daily News* reported that he was expected to keep the U of I presidency thanks to his "intellectual ability and capacity for getting things done."[42]

Unbeknownst to Stoddard, events were brewing in Chicago that eventually would lead to his undoing. At the center of those events was seemingly the unlikeliest of subjects: U of I vice president Andrew Ivy, the conscience of American science.

• • •

At first, the strange goings-on had nothing to do with Ivy or the U of I. In 1947, an Argentinian businessperson named Humberto Loretani became acquainted with two US counterparts, R. Edwin "Ed" Moore and Kenneth Brainard. Loretani represented a company called Duga that was based in Buenos Aires. The company was promoting "Kositerin," a new hypertension drug, and Duga was exploring whether there would be a market for it in the United States. Ed Moore was vice president of Bell and Gossett, a manufacturer of pumps and industrial equipment that was headquartered near Chicago and did business in Argentina. Moore was renowned for sales abilities that ranged well beyond pumps; he once sold a forty-car trainload of Smucker's apple butter to the Kroger grocery chain. "A doorbell never hurt any salesman's finger," he liked to say. Brainard was Moore's brother-in-law, and he had been president of the Beverly Hills Realty Board in California before he moved to Illinois.[43]

Moore and Brainard saw enough commercial potential in Kositerin to use their connections to set up meetings in the Chicago area about the new medicine. The star of the meetings would be the discoverer of the drug, Stevan Durovic, whom Loretani extolled as a genius. Durovic arrived in Chicago from Argentina in March 1949, and Moore and Brainard took him to the office of J. Roscoe Miller, dean of the Northwestern University Medical School, soon to be president of the entire university. The meeting came about through Moore's contacts with Nathan William MacChesney, a Northwestern alumnus and well-known attorney who, in the 1920s, had helped develop segregationist housing covenants in Chicago.[44]

A person attending the meeting later wrote a letter describing what had happened. Although the letter was unsigned, the author probably was an Argentinian visiting professor of medicine who was acting at the meeting as a translator. Durovic told the gathering in Miller's office that he was a Yugoslavian doctor who had been taken prisoner during the war and who subsequently received aid from the Vatican in finding refuge in Argentina. While doing research in that country, Durovic had discovered Kositerin, a minute dose of which cured high blood pressure. He claimed that he had successfully treated five thousand patients in Buenos Aires. "Everybody in the meeting held at the Dean's Office was convinced that Durovic was a quack," the letter writer recalled. "His talk was very much unscientific."

Even so, Miller indulged Durovic, which the letter writer speculated was because of the presence of Moore and Brainard, who "had helped occasionally the University in ways of endowments."[45]

In June and July of 1949, Northwestern doctors tested Kositerin on a handful of hypertensive cases at the university's medical facilities in downtown Chicago. The tests lasted only one week per patient and showed no benefits. Immediately afterward, one of the participating doctors, Fred W. Fitz, wrote to J. Roscoe Miller. Fitz indicated that he was "dismissing and filing in the archives of useless results the efforts on Kositerin." He noted that Durovic had refused to reveal the exact chemical structure of the drug, which immediately raised suspicions. Fitz added that "Durovic is not only unaware of the American methods of research and American physiological technics, but he is also either intellectually dishonest or stupid beyond my ken." The Northwestern doctor was worried that Durovic "may have pilfered some blank sheets of paper with our letterhead" and might use the stationery to embarrass the university in some way.[46]

Miller now faced the delicate task of getting rid of Durovic without angering university benefactors or influential alumni. He did so by sending Durovic and his two American sponsors to Andrew Ivy at the University of Illinois. It might have been a sincere effort to be helpful; Miller knew that Ivy was open to testing new substances. It also might have been intended as a light jab at Ivy, who three years earlier had left Northwestern for the U of I. Whatever his motivation, Miller could not possibly have imagined what would happen next.

Durovic arrived at Ivy's office along with Moore and Brainard.[47] Prior to their visit, Ivy had talked with Fred Fitz, who had told him about the negative test results with Kositerin; presumably, Fitz also had shared his personal opinion of Durovic. When Durovic told Ivy about Kositerin's supposed benefits while adding that the process of the drug's production was a business secret, Ivy displayed his customary scientific skepticism. "I advised [him] that the process should be revealed under the protection of a patent, since until that was done it would be very difficult to obtain professional acceptance in this country even though the material [might] prove to be of value," Ivy later recalled. The U of I vice president added that a secret remedy was highly unlikely to win acceptance from the Food and Drug Administration or the American Medical Association, nor could he ask for such a remedy to be studied in the U of I's facilities. However, as was again customary with Ivy, he agreed to test the drug on his own time outside the university to see if it had any "scientific and humanitarian" benefit.[48]

Durovic, Moore, and Brainard left Ivy's office. A short time later, in August 1949, they returned with a startling announcement—Durovic now had an entirely new drug that had yet to be named. Instead of treating hypertension, the new drug treated the most feared medical condition of all: cancer.

According to author Siddhartha Mukherjee, Americans in the late 1940s had reason to believe in "the potent and transformative capacity of science and technology," as exemplified by the development of penicillin and other antibiotics. Lethal diseases, including typhoid fever and tuberculosis, had been curbed. The glaring exception was cancer. As Mukherjee notes, "cancer still remained a black box, a mysterious entity that was best cut away en bloc rather than treated by some deeper medical insight." With chemotherapy still in its infancy, the only scientifically accepted therapies, with uncertain chances of success, were radiation and surgery: "a choice between the hot ray and the cold knife." Scientists and the lay public were eager to find alternatives to that stark, grim choice. "The process of growth is regular and orderly, held at an even tempo by some 'governor' which controls the speed of cell growth," wrote American Cancer Society president Frank E. Adair in the *New York Times Magazine* in 1946. "For fifty years, scientists have sought the answer to the mystery. What causes normal cells to revolt? What is the 'braking' power that ordinarily holds the cells in check?"[49]

Now, in Andrew Ivy's office in 1949, Stevan Durovic was suggesting that he had solved a major part of the mystery: he had discovered a governing or braking agent that would hold the cells in check. Durovic said that he had long hypothesized that living cells possessed such an agent. To test his hypothesis, he had obtained horses and a farm in Argentina where he had employed a means of stimulating the horses' reticuloendothelial system, which was associated with defense against disease. He then drew the horses' blood and used a chemical process to extract a substance that he injected into dogs and cats with cancer. The substance produced regressions in the animals' tumors. Durovic said that he had been working with two veterinarians at the University of Buenos Aires on this research; Humberto Loretani apparently knew nothing about it. Experiments with the new substance had continued in Argentina during Durovic's trip to the United States, and the reports continued to be good. It so happened that Durovic had brought some of the substance with him to Chicago. Rather than testing Kositerin (which Durovic surely realized would likely produce results similar to those obtained at Northwestern), Durovic wanted Ivy to test this new substance on cancer patients.

Ivy's interest was piqued in a way that it had not been concerning Kositerin. He was executive director of the National Advisory Cancer Council, and, in 1947, he had published an article in *Science* in which he asserted that "the rational approach to the secret of the cure of cancer" was to uncover the factors "responsible for limiting and regulating normal growth." In 1948, he had been forced to quash published rumors that he and a committee of doctors including Josiah J. Moore of the AMA were about to announce a cancer cure.[50]

Durovic's new anticancer substance seemed scientifically plausible to Ivy and consistent with his own theories on the regulation of cell growth. "I was reminded of the reports of Bogomolets on the antireticulocytotoxic serum [ACS] he produced," Ivy later said. Soviet scientist Aleksandr Bogomolets and his ACS drug had received extensive media attention in the 1940s. Bogomolets drew matter from the bone marrow of recently deceased people and injected it into horses; the horses were then bled and the ACS drug was extracted for human use. Some physicians and journalists had made what later would turn out to be wildly overstated claims for the drug. "This new 'elixir' almost miraculously builds up the body's resistance to cancer, preventing recurrence of tumors after the surgeon's knife has removed them the first time," declared a Johns Hopkins University doctor. ACS also was said to be effective against arthritis and to have the potential of extending the human life-span to 125 years or more. William Laurence, a *New York Times* science writer who had covered the first US atomic bomb test (and who later would be criticized for being a paid propagandist for the US government), asserted that Bogomolets's serum could be "a discovery more important to mankind than the atomic bomb." Henry Wachtel at Fordham University was doing related research with a lipid extracted from cattle pituitaries that he believed helped fight cancer.[51]

Ivy agreed to test Durovic's new drug, even though Durovic again refused to reveal the full details of how it was produced. For the time being, it was given the appropriately mysterious name of Substance X. Ivy worked with his longtime collaborator Louis Krasno in evaluating the medicine outside U of I facilities. Although initial tests on rats and mice showed that Substance X was not toxic, they also showed no anticancer activity. Disappointed but unsurprised, Ivy asked Krasno in late August 1949 to try the drug on two human patients with incurable cancer, fully expecting that their conditions would not change.

Soon after injecting the patients with the substance, Krasno excitedly phoned Ivy. "Either I have forgotten how to use a ruler, or else these cancers have gone down," Krasno reported. "You'd better come over and measure them for yourself."[52] Ivy confirmed that, indeed, the results seemed astonishing. Not only had the first patient's tumors shrunk, but also her pain had disappeared. The second patient, who had cancer of the tongue and jaw, had regained his ability to speak and eat solid food, again with a dramatic reduction in pain.

Intrigued, Ivy and Krasno added more cancer patients to the tests while recruiting help from another doctor, William F. P. Phillips, who was the personal physician to Ed Moore and Kenneth Brainard. The test results were promising enough that Ivy started dropping hints about Substance X in his public appearances. In an October 1949 talk titled "Cancer Research: Reasons for Hope," Ivy said that "the fact that a spontaneous regression of a cancer is known to occur and that they have occurred after the injection of certain substances convinces me that we may undoubtedly hope that a cure of cancer may in time be discovered."[53] The Chicago news media began hearing new rumors of a wondrous cancer drug at the U of I.

In February 1950, a new player appeared in Chicago: Marko Durovic. Like his brother Stevan, Marko had taken refuge in Argentina, where he had overseen Duga's business concerns. Now Marko was rejoining his brother in Chicago with what was said to be the remaining supply of Substance X. According to Humberto Loretani—who had remained behind in Buenos Aires—Marko was curtailing Duga's operations in Argentina, and Stevan had stopped communicating with his associates there. Loretani wrote to Ed Moore that the Durovics seemed intent on "severing all relations with all those persons" who had provided money to produce and promote Kositerin without receiving adequate compensation in return: "in other words, we all have fallen victims of the Durovic brothers." Loretani added that Marko "has shown a marked capacity for breaking down the reputation of those persons who do not accept his judgement and he is quite frightening in this respect."[54] On the basis of everything that had happened so far, Moore and Kenneth Brainard believed that they owned US distribution rights to Kositerin and also to Substance X; they had met Stevan at his arrival in Chicago and had accompanied him to the meetings that they personally had arranged for him while also doing him other favors. They now began detecting a distinct chill from the Durovic brothers—a slowly growing sense that any wealth that might be generated was not going to be shared.

Meanwhile, tests of the new drug continued to make Ivy and his associates believe that they might well be achieving a genuine breakthrough in cancer therapy. A Chicago doctor named John Pick administered the medicine to a Roman Catholic nun who had advanced cancer; she was said to display "spectacular improvement" for several days, and Columbus Hospital in Chicago allowed Pick to use the drug on additional terminal cancer patients. Pick's wife Marguerite, a prominent Chicago dressmaker, also was suffering from cancer that had spread to her liver and left her nearly comatose. She was injected with Substance X in November 1950, and Dr. Pick reported that she soon awoke and announced that she was hungry. After additional injections of the drug, Marguerite even left her sickbed and returned to work, but only briefly: she died in March 1951. "In retrospect, the patient should have received larger doses," Andrew Ivy would say of her.[55]

Eminent though he was, Ivy was not a cancer specialist. Neither was Louis Krasno, William Phillips, nor John Pick, the last of whom was best known for performing plastic surgery on inmates at Illinois's Stateville prison on the theory that improving physical appearance would reduce criminality. (A pulp detective magazine had published a story on Pick's work under the headline "New Mugs for Old Thugs.")[56] The doctors' lack of extensive clinical experience with cancer patients did not deter them, even if apparent beneficial effects from Substance X were only temporary. When the first patient whom Krasno had injected with the drug soon relapsed and died, Ivy blamed her death on a heart ailment rather than cancer. When the second patient treated by Krasno lost his jaw and died, the result was blamed on the patient's tumor having disintegrated so quickly. And, as with Marguerite Pick, negative results sometimes were attributed to the medicine not having been administered early enough or in high enough doses.

John Pick stayed committed to Substance X, but he seemed suspicious of the Durovics and apprehensive about the drug's future. In December 1950, he outlined his concerns to Ivy: they still did not know all the details of how the medicine was made or just how capable Stevan Durovic was; they also did not know what might happen in Argentina, where the drug had originated. Pick argued for establishing a means of producing Substance X in the Chicago area and for ensuring that Ivy retain scientific control over the drug. Pick said that his discussions with Stevan indicated that the Durovics wanted "*eventual and complete control of the marketing of the substance*." Moreover, Stevan asserted "that *he alone* is capable of following through [the production of the drug] *from beginning to end*." He also displayed "zealous anticipation of the 'open presentation' of substance 'X.' After that he 'knows *it will be easy* to do anything from raising money to research.'"[57]

Ivy again urged the Durovics to patent the drug and reveal exactly how it was produced. They replied that a patent would be too costly to protect, would not apply outside the United States, and would not prevent communists behind the Iron Curtain from getting hold of the substance. In early 1951, Ivy discovered that the Durovics—without consulting him first—had dissolved the entire supply of the drug in mineral oil and packaged it in ampules, which made it easy to distribute while also making it virtually impossible to analyze the drug chemically and determine precisely what it was. At that moment, Ivy nearly abandoned the whole project. He finally decided to continue his research on the medicine, believing that "we know too little about the biology of cancer to overlook any possibility." As for the secrecy surrounding Substance X, Ivy reasoned that he was "dealing with a business concern which had spent much money in the development of a product; none of the money had come from public sources. The business concern was unwilling to disclose until it had obtained the return of its investment, after which it was willing to reveal the process of production."[58]

Then US immigration authorities informed the Durovics that their visitor permits were expiring, and they soon would have to leave the country. If they left, any possibility of the drug being manufactured in the United States would vanish; so too would any possibility of Ivy continuing his work with the drug. The U of I vice president turned to powerful political friends. US senator Paul Douglas of Illinois agreed to sponsor a bill in Congress to grant the Durovics permanent resident status, but Douglas said that it would help the bill's chances if the new medicine were announced publicly. Ivy already was holding off reporters wanting to publish stories about the drug.

Ivy thus decided to hold a research presentation at Chicago's Drake Hotel on March 26, 1951. The presentation would outline the promising test results with the drug, which now had a new name—Krebiozen. Accounts of the origins of the name varied; it was said to have come from German words for "cancer" and "censor," or else it came from Greek words for "regulator of growth."[59] Apart from doctors, journalists, and fund raisers for cancer research, several elected officials were invited to the presentation: Douglas and fellow US senators Everett Dirksen of Illinois and Brien McMahon of Connecticut; Chicago mayor Martin Kennelly; president of the U of I Board of Trustees Park Livingston; and Cook County state's attorney John Boyle. Not invited were U of I president George Stoddard, U of I medical dean Stanley Olson, or U of I doctors thoroughly familiar with cancer research and treatment. Ivy later would say of Stoddard that "I didn't think he would be interested."[60]

John Boyle was extremely interested in Krebiozen. He had been elected state's attorney in Chicago in 1948 with the help of his publicist, a onetime reporter named John Pickering. Billboards across Cook County had displayed a stern-looking photo of Boyle next to the words "Gangsters Fear This Man." Pickering decided to promote Krebiozen by writing and sending a press release to the Chicago news media just prior to Ivy's research presentation. "The battle of medical science to find a cure for cancer achieved its realization today," the news release proclaimed. "Krebiozen is no longer a dream. Cancer need no longer signify certain and inevitable death. . . .

This dread disease has been genetically explained today and its successful cure has been realized."[61]

It was a grotesque overstatement of the facts, but it had the desired effect, at least presumably for Pickering: uninvited reporters descended on the Drake Hotel for Ivy's presentation. Ivy himself was appalled. He said that he knew nothing in advance about the news release. "I had to decide whether to ask the reporters to leave or to let them remain," he later recalled. "I decided it would be worse to drive them out than to let them stay. I felt like calling off the meeting, but decided that it would not be wise."

Ultimately, Ivy chose to plow ahead. He would, as he put it, "let nature take its course."[62] As he soon discovered, it was a course that led to chaos.

CHAPTER 2

Krebiozen Does Not Exist

In announcing Krebiozen to an audience of about one hundred people at the Drake Hotel, Andrew Ivy tried to limit the damage that the news release had inflicted in claiming a cancer cure. He said that he was issuing only a preliminary report based on observations of twenty-two people with late-stage cancer. He knew that the press already had been clamoring to print stories about the drug, and he hoped to preempt sensationalist news coverage that might raise false hopes. Krebiozen was not a cure, Ivy stressed, nor did it represent "the final goal in the chemotherapy of cancer." However, it was "an important step in that direction," and it offered "much promise in the management of the cancer patient." It therefore deserved careful clinical evaluation that doctors in attendance could help provide, although the drug at present was in very short supply. A brochure distributed at the presentation outlined the scientific theory behind Krebiozen and the results of the drug's tests on the twenty-two cancer cases. The brochure stated that twenty patients had "shown an improvement in their general condition" and "a regression of the cancer which has been consistent and has conformed to a general pattern." Although eight of the patients had subsequently died, the others were still alive, with five of them living a year or more after their first injections and two of them showing no cancer at all.[1]

Ivy succeeded in getting the newspapers to stop short of calling Krebiozen a cure, but they nonetheless heaped attention on the new drug. "The age-old search for a chemical bullet that will strike down cancer was believed by scientists to have come a step closer to success," the *Chicago Tribune* reported on its front page. One Illinois doctor said that Krebiozen could be "one of the greatest, if not the greatest" medical discoveries ever. After Ivy said that Stevan Durovic would not reveal how Krebiozen was produced because the communists had seized his property in Yugoslavia and he did not want them to get the drug, another doctor said that the new medicine "could be even more potent than the atomic bomb in deterring Russian aggression"; surely Stalin would want to "sit down and talk terms" to obtain Krebiozen for his people. A fund-raising appeal pointed to the medicine as a prime example of how investments in cancer research paid off: "The Miracle Drug Krebiozen Is a Direct Result!"[2]

Seemingly miraculous results from Krebiozen continued to occur. After the Drake Hotel announcement, Ivy and Durovic traveled to Michigan to administer the drug to US senator Arthur Vandenberg, who had terminal cancer. His doctor later reported that the senator "became more noticeably alert, and definitely manifested an appearance of well-being." Over the next couple of weeks, Vandenberg alternated periods of stupor with "days of uncanny revival during which he would read the paper, listen to the radio, watch television, smoke his beloved cigars, and converse freely and intelligently." The doctor attributed it all to Krebiozen, noting that although the senator did soon die, he did so without pain. Twelve-year-old Gary Cathcart of Wyoming also suffered from cancer, and Mayo Clinic doctors had told his family that they could do nothing more for him. After he received Krebiozen, his tumor was said to have dissolved completely. When the drug was stopped for a time, the tumor reappeared; when the drug was resumed in larger doses, the tumor shrank. Cathcart—who would grow up to become a Rhodes scholar—would be touted as one of Krebiozen's greatest success stories.[3]

However, not everything about Krebiozen was going according to plan, largely because there had not been much of a plan to begin with, according to Ivy. "We had no means to answer the extensive mail and telephone calls which obviously follows wide publicity," he later said. "No organization had been established. In fact, none had been discussed." Although a University of Illinois public relations officer was present at the Drake Hotel announcement, the U of I still was blindsided by an estimated eleven thousand phone calls and messages from around the world inquiring about and begging for Krebiozen. A few individuals received the drug, including a dying Brazilian physician in Rio de Janeiro and a dying woman in Delaware, the latter being administered the medicine following a mercy flight from Chicago. Most other people failed in their attempts to get Krebiozen, no matter how desperate their pleas. One Massachusetts woman vowed that she would hitchhike to Chicago to obtain the drug for her terminally ill child. In response to such heartbreaking stories, U of I representatives could offer little consolation. "Do not come to Chicago," was their standard message. "Remain at home until clinical study and evaluation of the serum is completed."[4]

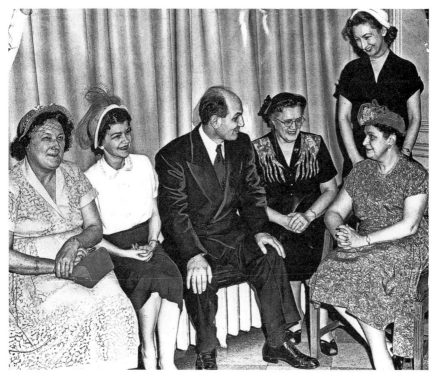

Stevan Durovic at the March 1951 announcement of Krebiozen at Chicago's Drake Hotel. Durovic was photographed with women who said that they had benefited from the drug. (Chicago Tribune/TCA)

The Krebiozen presentation had been called partly to keep Stevan Durovic and his brother Marko in the United States, and in that respect the presentation succeeded. US senator Paul Douglas eventually helped get them permanent resident status, although that process would take another year to complete.[5] The press found the brothers intriguing. Stevan was described as a "little sharp-faced, bald-headed man who for 20 years has so immersed himself in research that he has to be reminded to buy new socks and who hasn't bothered to get a new hat in the last nine years"; his older brother Marko was "a dark, sleek, impeccably groomed Yugoslavian lawyer" of considerable means.[6] The *Chicago Tribune* published a five-part series relating the Durovics' dramatic life story. They were said to be sons of a high-ranking public official in Montenegro. Stevan studied at the Sorbonne in Paris before earning his medical degree and becoming a professor of medicine in Belgrade. Marko, who had served as a judge as well as an attorney, made his fortune through a munitions company and other business enterprises. Stevan was conscripted into the Yugoslav military during World War II and was captured and sent to an Italian prison camp. Through the intercession of Italy's Queen Elena, who originally was from Montenegro, Stevan was released; and with the personal assistance of Pope Pius XII, the two brothers traveled via Spain to the neutral country of Argentina in 1942. There, Stevan made his scientific breakthroughs underwritten by Marko's money.[7]

The Durovics' story seemed in some ways similar to the stories of other wartime European émigrés whose scientific expertise was now benefiting the United States. But the mystery surrounding the Durovics was unusually thick. One observer suggested that "central casting would have placed them in a counter-espionage vehicle, slipping on and off the Orient Express."[8] Some news coverage of them hinted at unsavory doings, with Kositerin—which had not been mentioned at all at the Drake Hotel—quickly coming to light. Northwestern University's Fred Fitz and J. Roscoe Miller told the Chicago newspapers of the negative test results two years earlier with the alleged hypertension medication. Both men also distinctly remembered that Stevan Durovic had said that Kositerin was derived from horse blood, just as Krebiozen was supposed to be. Could the striking similarities in the two drugs' names and origins be a coincidence?

At first, Stevan told the press that he knew nothing about Kositerin; he then reversed himself and blamed his confusion on his difficulties with English. Kositerin and Krebiozen were in fact two different drugs, he would say, and Kositerin came from cattle blood rather than horse blood. Stevan said that he had come to the United States expressly to meet Andrew Ivy and get Krebiozen tested on people with cancer. However, when Ed Moore and Kenneth Brainard met him at the airport and took him to Miller's office at Northwestern, Stevan decided to present his hypertension drug instead, because Miller was a heart specialist. Only when Stevan finally met Ivy did he reveal the existence of Krebiozen. Stevan's explanation did not exactly align with Ivy's recollection, which was that the first meeting between the two men discussed only Kositerin; the cancer medicine was not mentioned until their second meeting. Either way, suspicions persisted that Kositerin and Krebiozen were one and the same.[9]

Also coming to light were the escalating conflicts between the Durovic brothers and Moore and Brainard, who had attended the Drake Hotel announcement and spoken to reporters afterward. "We were selected to aid Dr. Durovic's institute in bringing about such things as happened today on the idea that this might develop into something very interesting and profitable," Brainard had told the reporters. Suddenly, Marko elbowed his way into the discussion to announce grimly that his brother had no connection to the two Americans. Furthermore, according to Marko, there had been sinister efforts to separate him from Stevan and send him back to

Argentina. Stevan said that he and his brother were the victims of "intrigue and selfish interests."[10]

The Durovic brothers were at odds with Ivy and his associates as well, although those tensions would not become public for some time. Ivy had helped set up a nonprofit organization called the Krebiozen Research Foundation to deflect criticism that the drug was primarily a moneymaking venture. Yet the Durovics made it clear that they expected money. One of the foundation's directors was Cook County state's attorney John Boyle, whose publicist had proclaimed Krebiozen to be a cancer cure; Boyle also had urged Paul Douglas to help the Durovics get permanent residency. The brothers asked Boyle where they could get three million dollars, which they said would go toward building a Krebiozen production plant in the United States. John Pick, the doctor who already had expressed his uneasiness about the Durovics to Ivy, told the brothers that no bank would lend them a large sum of money for a drug about which so little was known. The Eli Lilly pharmaceutical company made a $1.1 million offer to obtain rights to Krebiozen, contingent on the Durovics patenting the formula and means of production while also permitting the company to test the medicine for safety and efficacy. When Stevan instead proposed manufacturing the drug himself, with Eli Lilly allowed only to distribute it with no questions asked, the company quickly withdrew its offer.[11]

It was decided that the Krebiozen Research Foundation would acquire the existing supply of Krebiozen and pay back the Durovics through the resale of the drug, if the foundation could successfully navigate federal drug regulations and also receive favorable tax rulings from the US Department of the Treasury. The Durovics said that they had spent more than $1.3 million in developing the medicine, and they and the foundation wanted to claim that sum as a nontaxable business expense. After the government asked for much more information, including documentation of the Durovics' expenditures, the foundation changed its request: it now wanted to claim Krebiozen as a capital asset, with any profits from its sale ruled as a long-term capital gain. That request was complicated by the fact that the Durovics had paid no duty on the drug when they brought it into the United States, making it harder to claim it as highly valuable property. A Texas lawyer proposed that the Durovics sell the drug to the foundation in Bermuda, where they would not have to pay US income taxes. Senator Douglas—who was advising the foundation—dismissed that idea as "fishy." He told the Durovics that "were it not for Dr. Ivy, I would be very skeptical of the whole damn [Krebiozen] thing," and he pleaded with them not to "allow anything to happen which might reflect upon this man's reputation, integrity, and standing as a scientist."[12]

Ivy himself was worried, according to the minutes from a foundation meeting in June 1951. The Durovics were threatening to leave the United States and take Krebiozen with them. Pick angrily told them that "if you fail with our help to put Krebiozen over in this country, you will be finished the world over." Ivy then jumped into the exchange. "There are too many people already who do not [just] think but [also] say that I and Dr. Pick are a couple of saps," Ivy said. "Were I to speak further and from a purely selfish standpoint, I should tell you right now that both Dr. Pick and I would have been better off had we never laid eyes on you." Adding that he had committed to Krebiozen purely in hopes of giving people with cancer a new treatment option, Ivy informed the Durovics that "from now on you will do what I tell you," even though the brothers to that point had shown little inclination to do what anyone else said.[13]

Ivy was correct in saying that many people viewed him as a sap; they had done so starting from the first minutes of the Drake Hotel presentation. Invited doctors who arrived at the hotel were greeted by the sight of John Pickering—the state's attorney publicist—handing out promotional photographs and press releases, which prompted many of the doctors to turn around and leave. Later, Ivy marched out a group of women who had taken and apparently prospered with Krebiozen. Although some of the doctors who had stayed for the presentation applauded, others left. Private meetings to announce scientific results and raise research funds were not uncommon, but this meeting had an air of hoopla and hucksterism about it that seemed distinctly unscientific. The most accepted means of presenting such a research report was through a peer-reviewed medical journal, which Ivy said he had eschewed because the Durovics did not want to reveal the process of producing Krebiozen. Many scientists and doctors found that excuse especially egregious. "Never have I experienced so much unfavorable comment on the part of the profession as has been my experience as the result of the introduction of Krebiozen," one Illinois doctor wrote to Ivy in April 1951. In fact, the National Advisory Cancer Council, which Ivy had served as executive director, explicitly said that secrecy of any kind about the nature or composition of a cancer treatment was unethical.[14]

The ethical concerns were amplified in an editorial the following month in the *Proceedings of the Institute of Medicine of Chicago*. "Accepted requirements for medical reporting have developed because of the importance of protecting the profession and the public from false or misleading claims," the editorial said. "Violation of these requirements, as the krebiozen incident demonstrates, has unfortunate consequences in arousing false hopes which tend to discredit the medical profession. Such a regrettable disregard for the established practice cannot be condoned."[15]

What of Krebiozen's apparently amazing results? The week after the Drake Hotel presentation, one skeptical observer wrote that reports about the drug were "like a hundred others" purporting breakthroughs in cancer treatment: "But after a thousand or so cases of cancer on which the new, strange substances have been tried are analyzed, it turns out that nothing more than relief of pain and temporary regressions of tumors have been achieved." Another observer pointed out that injections of many substances, even milk or vegetable broth, could trigger a brief immune reaction against the inflammation surrounding malignant tumors without otherwise affecting cancer in any way.[16] Doctors and scientists over the years have consistently said that testimonials about a drug's alleged benefits are no substitute for scientific evidence. Phony remedies might temporarily seem to work for a host of reasons: the disease already might have run its course or be cyclical in nature, the placebo effect might be at play, the patient might also have been treated with mainstream medicines that have produced positive effects, and so forth. Regardless, the phony remedies are not really curing anything.[17]

The American Medical Association (AMA), which is headquartered in Chicago, was the biggest skeptic of all concerning Krebiozen. Morris Fishbein, a longtime AMA leader, blasted the secrecy about the drug: "Secrecy is associated with attempts to conceal lack of merit." AMA representatives Norman DeNosaquo and Oliver Field had attended the Drake Hotel presentation; Field was the association's director of investigation in potential health-fraud cases, and DeNosaquo was tasked with writing a summary of the event for the AMA's files. When Ivy offered attendees free samples of the drug for testing purposes, DeNosaquo reported that "people were grabbing them like you would expect your wife to grab 52-gauge nylon hose at 49 cents a pair." DeNosaquo made little effort to hide his disdain during the presentation. People sitting near him heard him muttering: "Ivy, you goddamned quack."[18]

With the AMA determined to prove that Krebiozen was quackery—and Ivy equally determined not to be crucified for his belief in Krebiozen[19]—the simmering debate over the drug would turn extraordinarily bitter.

• • •

The AMA had long been at the forefront of the battle against medical quackery. Starting in the early twentieth century, the organization regularly published exposés of patent medicines and crooked doctors in the influential *Journal of the American Medical Association* (*JAMA*), which Morris Fishbein edited; Fishbein had led the fight to expose the notorious health fraudster John Brinkley. The AMA also served as the primary clearinghouse for people seeking information about quackery. "No other organization in the nation after 1906 remotely rivaled the AMA in exposing the graft and ravages of the nostrum vendors," a history of the AMA would note, adding that "the ghouls of cancer quackery" were particular targets of the association's wrath.[20]

Although the AMA's work in that field was justly celebrated, the organization also had become highly controversial by the time that Krebiozen emerged in 1951. Under Fishbein's leadership, it had grown into what journalist Milton Mayer described as "the most terrifying trade organization on earth." Doctors who did not toe the AMA's line risked expulsion, which Mayer said was "a doctor's death warrant." Doctors who did toe the line were rewarded by an association that zealously promoted their financial interests, in part by limiting the supply of medical providers and services. The AMA's critics said that the organization exerted its enormous power to restrict medical school enrollment and the expansion of health-care facilities.[21]

In particular, the AMA waged war against group health insurance programs. Mayer suggested that this multimillion-dollar campaign was literally the most terrifying thing about the organization: it sought to "terrify [the doctor] into terrifying his patients into terrifying their Congressmen to vote against 'socialized medicine.'" The campaign had started early in the Depression when a national committee highlighted the chronic structural inequities in US health care and recommended alternatives that included group insurance plans. Fishbein charged that the committee's recommendations pitted "Americanism versus sovietism" and threatened to deprive each citizen of the fundamental "right to pick his own doctor and his own hospital." The AMA's battle to prevent doctors from participating in prepaid, low-cost health groups grew so ferocious that the US government launched an antitrust suit against the organization, which the AMA lost in 1943. Fishbein acknowledged that the suit's outcome served "to convict the AMA in the eyes of the people as being a predatory, antisocial monopoly." Even so, the AMA still led a successful fight after World War II to block President Harry Truman's national health insurance proposals, although concerns over Fishbein's leadership grew to the point that he was ousted from the organization's staff in 1949.[22]

Krebiozen had been on the AMA's quackery radar since early 1950, when reports to the association's offices indicated that Dr. William Phillips was injecting patients with a serum that was being promoted as a cancer cure.[23] After the AMA's representatives attended the Drake Hotel announcement in March 1951, the organization began looking into the drug more systematically. In May AMA treasurer Josiah J. "JJ" Moore asked Dr. Peter Neskow to accompany him to a meeting with the Durovic brothers, with Neskow serving as interpreter. Also present were Oliver Field and Paul Wermer of the AMA's Committee on Research. According to an affidavit that Neskow later gave, the meeting began cordially enough. Field asked Stevan about the chemical nature of Krebiozen, and Stevan politely parried the query by saying that the secret behind the drug would be revealed in due course—but not quite yet.

Then, according to Neskow, JJ Moore asked the brothers whether they had a contract with Ed Moore (who was unrelated to JJ) and Kenneth Brainard to distribute Krebiozen. When Stevan denied the existence of any such contract, the AMA treasurer told the Durovics that they "must give the distribution of Krebiozen" to the two Americans. Marko leaped to his feet. "Stop!" he shouted in English, pronouncing the word with a long o like "soap." Heatedly continuing in his native tongue, he said that if the AMA representatives were interested purely in the science behind Krebiozen, the Durovics would give them their complete cooperation. However, if they were probing into the brothers' private business affairs (and here again Marko switched to English with the long o), "stop!"—the Durovics would not permit such effrontery. Neskow recalled that the "atmosphere became very tense and unpleasant," with JJ Moore sardonically complimenting Marko for being such a "fine and sharp lawyer." Ivy did not attend the meeting, but he later would remember that it was about this time that he started hearing that Moore, with whom he previously had worked on cancer research, was "out to get" him. In July 1951, the AMA revealed that it had launched a full-fledged critical study of Krebiozen, with the results to be announced by the fall.[24]

Some of Ivy's closest scientific colleagues had become deeply concerned. Franklin Bing had worked for many years as an AMA researcher. He urged Ivy to meet with him, with Ivy's University of Chicago mentor Anton J. Carlson, and with Ivy's former Northwestern University colleague Smith Freeman. The three men wanted to review Ivy's Krebiozen data. "I believe it is imperative that we look over the evidence available to you, at the earliest possible moment, to determine whether we can concur in your interpretation of the material," Bing wrote to Ivy early that summer. Carlson, the legendary physiologist who always demanded to see the evidence backing scientific claims, wrote to Ivy as well. "We in science cannot under any circumstances depart from ethics," Carlson said scoldingly. "It was up to you, you had the power, why did you not exclude the newspaper reporters from your [Drake Hotel] meeting? . . . How extensive and reliable was the evidence for Krebiozen? Why was a preliminary report by you in a medical journal considered inadequate?" Carlson signed his letter "your troubled friend."[25]

Such entreaties did not move Ivy. On August 1, Bing wrote to him again. Bing had learned that the AMA was wrapping up its study of one hundred patients who had received Krebiozen, "and in absolutely 100% of these cases there is no clear cut evidence to permit a conclusion that Krebiozen is of any value in the treatment of cancer." Bing told Ivy that he had "entered this affair not only with an open mind, but one which was prejudiced in your favor. How else could I be after all of these years of association and the kindnesses with which you have favored me on numerous occasions?" However, he feared that the AMA report would result in the Chicago Medical Society declaring that Ivy was no longer a member in good standing and also in the U of I stripping Ivy of his administrative post. "When the American Medical Association's support fails, you will be ruined as completely and thoroughly as any man can possibly be ruined," Bing wrote. "When that report of the AMA appears, you're sunk, and you and your family will suffer and every good cause for which you have fought will suffer also." He begged Ivy to renounce Krebiozen before it was too late.[26]

Ivy responded to Bing promptly and warmly, but also negatively. "I cannot bring myself to believe that Krebiozen is an inert substance in the cancer patient," Ivy told him. "No one knows better than you that you can't break faith with yourself and that you must let your conscience and belief in what you think is right be your guide. On this basis I am willing and ready to take the consequences, whatever they might be." Bing wrote to Ivy twice more in August pleading with him to change his mind, telling him that "you have been associating with the wrong kind of people lately," but it was to no avail.[27]

In September, *Science* magazine published a commentary from oncologist Cornelius P. Rhoads on Krebiozen. Noting that "the history of the search for better means of cancer control is littered with the hidden wrecks of premature announcements based upon unwarranted conclusions," Rhoads argued that the evidence concerning Krebiozen made it impossible "to conclude that it is capable of exerting salutary effect on the course of neoplastic disease in man." In a response published alongside Rhoads's commentary, Ivy said simply that he continued to believe "that the substance merits further careful clinical investigation." That same month, a *New England Journal of Medicine* editorial dismissed Krebiozen and Ivy without mentioning them by name. The journal said that much-ballyhooed cancer drugs that "fail to live up to the publicity that is accorded them may cause as many heartaches as the out-and-out frauds that are perpetrated on the public." It added that the impetus behind such drugs often stemmed from "a mixture of egoism and enthusiasm in some scientifically myopic person."[28]

No doubt anticipating that whatever was about to come from the AMA would likely be even more damning, Stevan Durovic wrote to the organization to try to forestall its report on Krebiozen. He said that the drug was being distributed free of charge for tests on more than four hundred patients in some one hundred clinics in the United States and fifteen countries overseas. "We are seriously concerned that a report now would impede the progress of our investigation," Durovic said, adding that it "would be of distinct disadvantage for the cancer patient." Durovic tried to dispel Krebiozen's stigma of secrecy by offering to reveal his method of stimulating horses' reticuloendothelial systems (it later was said to be an injection of the *Actinomyces bovis* bacterium that caused a condition called lumpy jaw in the animals). In his own communication to the AMA, John Pick said that Durovic's gesture indicated that Krebiozen's production process was "not a secret in the absolute sense of the word." However, nothing else about the process was revealed.[29]

Durovic's and Pick's efforts to placate the AMA were for naught. In October, the organization published its Krebiozen report in *JAMA*. The report said that normally the association would not bother trying to evaluate the clinical effects of a substance of such obscure origins, but "the importunities of physicians for authentic information and the tremendous worldwide public interest created a moral obligation to the profession and to the laity which transcended the issue of medical ethics ordinarily applicable to secret remedies." The AMA's Committee on Research had obtained one hundred Krebiozen case studies from across the country, including the U of I's tumor clinic. A group of cancer experts from Chicago-area medical schools (excluding the U of I) then examined the case studies. "Not one of the patients observed has shown any appreciable alteration in the course of the primary tumor growth, although two patients showed equivocal, temporary response," said the report. Forty-four patients had died. The report noted that subjective patient responses were notoriously unreliable, as shown by a recent study of people with terminal cancer who had received cortisone: they had displayed "a remarkable feeling of well-being and strength accompanied by relative freedom from pain and increased appetite and ambulation which persisted to practically the day of death." But, in fact, they had died; their cancer had not abated. Temporary regression of a metastatic lesion was not a cure. "The public must be dissuaded of the belief that all forms of cancer represent a single disease which progresses in the same manner, by the same course, and responds uniformly to therapy," the report declared. In conclusion, it said that its findings had failed to confirm Ivy's claims for Krebiozen.[30]

The AMA report made news across the country. The *Washington Post* called the report "an utterly demolishing broadside." A *Chicago Tribune* editorial was especially scathing: "Medically speaking, krebiozen is dead. It should be buried without ceremony. If there are any attempts to use it commercially, or to dismiss the findings of the A. M. A. as motivated by 'the jealousy of the medical trust'—a pet phrase of every cancer quack in the land—State's Attorney Boyle should take the matter up with the grand jury. He already has evidenced an interest in krebiozen rather unusual in a layman."[31]

Concurrent with the AMA report, a committee of cancer experts from the National Research Council also pronounced Krebiozen worthless. In November, much as Franklin Bing had predicted some months earlier, the Chicago Medical Society found Ivy guilty of unethical conduct and suspended him for three months. Ivy responded that he was not guilty of a breach of ethics—he was not profiting financially from Krebiozen, which was not being sold—but he indicated that he would not appeal the society's decision. As for the AMA, Ivy again asserted that his personal observations of Krebiozen patients had convinced him that the drug warranted serious study. "Were that not so, I would not be contributing an average of six hours of my time every day to its investigation," he said. "The current publicity is particularly unfortunate because time has not permitted a complete analysis of reports on more than 600 patients, many of whom have received larger doses than the earlier patients."[32]

Ivy could not believe that the AMA would negate what seemed to him to be perfectly legitimate and potentially trailblazing research. From the start, the Durovic brothers had been murmuring darkly about a conspiracy. Their onetime business associate Humberto Loretani had come to Chicago from Argentina earlier that year and had met with Ivy as well as JJ Moore and Paul Wermer of the AMA. The men had tried to convince Ivy that the Durovics were not to be trusted. Yet the Durovics said that they, too, had met with Loretani with Ivy not present, and Loretani had told them that if they did not hand over the rights to Krebiozen to Ed Moore and Kenneth Brainard, the AMA and JJ Moore would destroy them. The Durovics also claimed that Loretani had told them that a payoff of $2.5 million would make the AMA investigation go away. Ivy began wondering whether this hair-raising tale might actually be true: as he put it, "that someone or some group of persons was out to destroy Krebiozen and to sabotage research on the substance" and "that the destruction of A. C. Ivy was in the picture." Ivy also wondered whether Franklin Bing's letter that warned of professional ruin if he did not drop Krebiozen had been intended to intimidate him—do what the AMA tells you or face the consequences.[33]

Ivy at least could take comfort in the fact that one of Bing's predictions had yet to transpire: he still held his administrative position at the U of I. Indeed, the university was publicly backing him. "We want no quarrel with the A. M. A.," said U of I Board of Trustees president Park Livingston.

"However, the board has great confidence in Dr. Ivy as a man looking for evidence."[34] Soon enough, though, the university would start looking for its own evidence, and the confidence of one key individual—the university president—would start to crumble.

• • •

Unlike Livingston, George Stoddard had not been invited to the Drake Hotel Krebiozen announcement in March 1951; the U of I president learned about the drug for the first time through the news media. Provost Coleman Griffith also had known nothing in advance. According to Griffith, Stoddard told him that Ivy's method of making the announcement "was a strange and unusual way of doing university business but, if Doctor Ivy really had something, it would be a great day for the University of Illinois." Certainly, it seemed like a welcome piece of upbeat news following so much turmoil over the College of Commerce and other university units. Stoddard and Griffith met with Ivy a couple of times over the next few months after the Krebiozen announcement. Griffith remembered "a somewhat vague referenc[e] by Doctor Ivy to certain interferences from outside the University, but Doctor Ivy assured me that these were of no concern to me."[35]

Then came the AMA's negative report on Krebiozen and the Chicago Medical Society's suspension of Ivy. Stoddard stood by his vice president, just as Livingston had. The U of I president told the press that he would confer with Ivy about making further investigations of Krebiozen to try to confirm the drug's efficacy. Ivy had submitted an undated letter of resignation upon taking the U of I vice presidency; he said that he routinely gave his employers such a letter to allow them to dismiss him easily should they deem it necessary. "I would never act upon that kind of a resignation as a matter of principle," Stoddard said to the press. "I don't believe in a sword dangling over a man's head. If anyone asks me if I am asking for Doctor Ivy's resignation, the answer is no."[36]

Livingston was delighted by Stoddard's stance. "For the first time since he became president, George has behaved like a university president," Livingston told Griffith. The provost noted that Livingston showed an "avid interest in Krebiozen" to the point of actively trying to resolve the dispute between the Durovic brothers and Ed Moore and Kenneth Brainard. "I gained the clear impression that Mr. Livingston was eager to secure support for Doctor Ivy," Griffith recalled. But other university trustees were concerned about Ivy's suspension from the medical society; they believed that it reflected negatively on the U of I. Privately, Stoddard and Griffith felt the same way. The university president was coming under fire from doctors in Champaign-Urbana, home of the main campus. The Champaign County

Medical Society criticized Stoddard for having "not kept faith with the high ideals of the university. Nor has he discharged a solemn obligation to the citizens of Illinois when he failed to publicly rebuke Dr. Ivy for seeking credit rather than results, and proclaiming an empty falsehood instead of the truth."[37]

On the other hand, Stoddard also had recently received a letter from Warren Cole, a U of I medical professor who eventually would serve as president of the American Cancer Society. Cole acknowledged the negative reaction from doctors and scientists to Ivy's involvement with Krebiozen. "Counterbalancing this reaction is the reaction of the public at large, which is a great admirer of Dr. Ivy," Cole wrote to Stoddard. "I think we should also include the members of the State Legislature in this group." Stoddard, of course, already had drawn the ire of a number of Illinois legislators. Cole therefore advised that the university not act too hastily against Ivy, lest it appear that the U of I was being unduly influenced by the AMA or the Chicago Medical Society.[38]

Caught in the middle of the Krebiozen dispute was U of I medical dean Stanley Olson. No one understood better than he the dangers of alienating powerful public officials. He had become dean just one year previously to replace John Youmans, who had resigned after falling afoul of state lawmakers who were unhappy that preference was not being given to local applicants for admissions to the university's medical school and jobs in the university's offices and clinics. Olson also understood that Ivy's fundraising prowess had greatly benefited the U of I's medical programs and that Ivy enjoyed strong support from many members of the medical faculty. Earlier in 1951, Illinois governor Adlai Stevenson had added to Ivy's power by appointing him to the Medical Center Commission in Chicago. The commission oversaw the physical development of the city's West Side medical facilities, which included the U of I's hospital as well as the Cook County Hospital and the Presbyterian Hospital (later known as the Rush University Medical Center). The commission's support was essential for the future expansion of the U of I's medical programs.[39]

Those programs' reputation rested on more than just new buildings, however; increasingly, it also would depend on research. Although US government laboratories had conducted a significant amount of medical research during World War II, by the early 1950s such research had begun shifting to university-based medical schools, with the government supporting the work through grants and contracts. Universities viewed that change with some apprehension about whether it would distort their educational mission and increase their dependence on the federal government. Nevertheless, the 1950s would see the rapid rise of what would be called the federal grant university, with the U of I becoming a prime beneficiary of government money. The National Institutes of Health, of which the National Cancer Institute was a part, would be one of the biggest underwriters of university research, deciding what to fund through a scientific peer-review system that tended to favor well-established, noncontroversial lines of inquiry.[40]

By hiring Ivy, the U of I had sought to enhance its standing in medical research. Along with creating the vice president position to lure him from Northwestern, the U of I also had created an academic unit for him: the Department of Clinical Science, whose goal was said to be "the union of all branches of medical science" in seeking "to define and to advance knowledge regarding disease." The unit originally was to be called the Department of Experimental Medicine, but some U of I medical faculty objected. They believed that the name might give the mistaken impression that the only scientific experimentation taking place in the university's medical programs was in that single department, whereas, in fact, a substantial program of such research was already underway.[41]

Now, the U of I's research reputation was being undermined by Ivy. He was part of an older generation of researchers who could dabble in whatever interested them and did not have to rely so heavily on government funding. Stevan Durovic had come to the United States to try to entice a university's interest in his medicines; he recognized the prestige that endorsement from a major university medical program could bring him. Improbably, he had managed to garner Ivy's support for Krebiozen. When Ivy announced the drug at the Drake Hotel, he had attracted intense attention from patients, politicians, businesspeople, and other individuals with no direct connection to science or academia—part of the external sets of interests that would increasingly confront the postwar "multiversity."[42] The peer-review system, which could have prevented the Krebiozen imbroglio by promptly squelching research on the dubious medication, had instead been bypassed completely, and now scientists' efforts to stop the drug faced fierce political resistance. Making matters worse was an administrative oddity that had not been foreseen by U of I officials when they recruited Ivy. In creating the Department of Clinical Science with Ivy as its head, the university made Ivy report to Olson, the medical dean. At the same time, in making Ivy vice president in charge of the Chicago medical programs, the university made Olson report to Ivy. In short, Ivy and Olson were simultaneously each other's superior and subordinate, putting Olson in a virtually impossible position in trying to deal with Krebiozen.

Olson outlined his frustrations in a letter to President Stoddard in November 1951, soon after the Chicago Medical Society suspended Ivy. "The lack of administrative restraint upon a member of the faculty who is also the chief administrative officer on the Chicago Professional Colleges campus is easily explained," said Olson. "I am not at all sure, however, that this fact relieves me as dean of the College of Medicine of all responsibility." Olson made it clear to Stoddard that he believed that Ivy was in over his head in undertaking complicated clinical research with Krebiozen: "While Doctor Ivy's abilities are outstanding, his clinical experience has been sporadic and incidental to his work as a physiologist and would not qualify him for a faculty position in any of the clinical departments of the College of Medicine." Ivy was refusing to consult with U of I colleagues more experienced in those matters. He had ignored basic scientific protocol in reporting his results, and he was depending heavily on unreliable survey data from doctors who had administered Krebiozen to patients whom Ivy had never personally seen. "This whole affair has been extremely distasteful to the faculty of the College of Medicine," Olson told Stoddard, adding that "persons in academic positions at many institutions are gravely concerned and are looking to see what position the University will take."[43]

Stoddard thus faced a serious dilemma in deciding how to proceed. He consulted with the U of I Board of Trustees at its November meeting in Chicago. The trustees agreed with Stoddard that Krebiozen was an administrative matter: that is, they granted the university president the authority to determine a course of action. Stoddard, believing that the U of I needed to make its own independent assessment, told the trustees that he wanted "to determine definitely the value of the drug under research and clinical conditions" and "to validate to the satisfaction of all concerned the effects of Krebiozen on cancer patients." To that end, he appointed a research validation committee. Warren Cole—the U of I medical professor who had urged caution in the Krebiozen matter—would head the committee, which would include five other doctors drawn from the U of I and other universities. Ivy agreed to all the proposed members except for Danely Slaughter, whose U of I Tumor Clinic had supplied many of the cases that the AMA included in its critical Krebiozen report. Slaughter was replaced with a different doctor on what became known as the Cole Committee. Stoddard asked the committee to analyze Ivy's research results, while Ivy was given a leave of absence in January and February of 1952 to examine the several hundred new Krebiozen case studies that he said he had amassed. He then was supposed to report his findings to the committee.[44]

It took Ivy until June to submit his report. He had hoped to include a chemical analysis of Krebiozen, but the Durovics' preemptive move to dissolve the drug in mineral oil and seal it in glass ampules made such an analysis exceptionally difficult. A microanalytical laboratory ended up

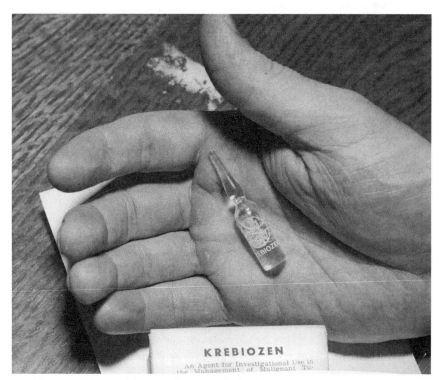

Krebiozen as it would most frequently be distributed—in tiny glass ampules for what was called "investigational use." What actually was in the ampules would remain a mystery. (STM-036541597, Chicago Sun-Times Collection, Chicago History Museum)

inadvertently crushing the glass together with the printed labels, the oil, and whatever else might be in the ampules. So there was nothing in Ivy's report to the Cole Committee to clear up the mystery of what the drug actually might be.[45]

Still, the report was measuredly enthusiastic. According to Ivy, it could not be said for certain that Krebiozen prolonged life or had an antitumor effect. But the drug did demonstrate definite biological activity with both objective and subjective improvements in people with cancer. A little more than half of the patients in his study had shown a decrease in tumor size, and more than two-thirds of them had reported a decrease in pain. Soon after issuing his report to the U of I, Ivy received encouraging accounts from Marquette University in Milwaukee and from Lankenau Hospital in Philadelphia about their experiments with Krebiozen. A Marquette doctor had treated two patients with the drug. The first patient showed a decrease in pain and a gain in weight (although she also had received hormone and radiation therapy); the second patient demonstrated symptomatic improvement for several months. Lankenau reported that the hospital's treatment of forty patients with Krebiozen showed that the drug "definitely has a biological effect on tumor cells in the human," with a few cases showing "complete disappearance of metastatic lesions."[46]

The Cole Committee reviewed Ivy's case studies along with some of Lankenau's patient studies. The committee worked under tight time pressure with the unenviable assignment of validating or invalidating a renowned scientist's research results. In addition, the committee was headed by a U of I doctor who worked under Ivy's administrative oversight and who was acutely conscious of the potential political ramifications of Krebiozen. Perhaps for those reasons, the Cole Committee's report to President Stoddard in September 1952 was notably mealymouthed. "We have found no acceptable evidence that any malignant tumor has been cured and none has been claimed in Dr. Ivy's report," the committee said. "We have found in the evidence submitted no evidence that prolongation of life has been effected and no claim in this direction has been made in Dr. Ivy's report." Ivy had presented no evidence that Krebiozen "produced degenerative or regressive changes in tumor cells, and no unequivocal oncolytic effect is claimed in his report." The committee also had found no conclusive evidence that the medicine could make metastatic lesions disappear, nor did it believe that Krebiozen cured cancer—but, again, Ivy had made no such definitive claims about the drug. On the other hand, said the committee, "we cannot state that it is entirely devoid of biological activity."[47]

The Cole Committee did make one thing clear: the secrecy surrounding Krebiozen's composition and preparation could not continue. "In our opinion it would be inconclusive if not futile to conduct further clinical investigation unless it is first possible to dispel the mystery which surrounds the nature of the material," the committee report said. "In default of this step no further consideration should be given to the problem." If, however, the mystery finally were dispelled, the committee recommended further clinical investigation of Krebiozen. The investigation should include adequate animal testing for both safety and efficacy (which Ivy had not done to that point), as well as adequate control groups to compare patients who received the medicine with patients who did not receive it (which Ivy also had not done to that point). That way, Krebiozen's value or lack thereof could be determined conclusively.[48]

Whatever its hedging, the Cole Committee hardly seemed to view Krebiozen as a potential wonder drug, having focused on everything that the drug had *not* been shown to do. The press viewed the committee's report in that light. "A research committee of six nationally known medical experts has completed a report rejecting any claims of beneficial results made for krebiozen," the *Chicago Tribune* reported in a front-page story. The newspaper also noted that the committee's examination of case studies at Lankenau Hospital did not support suggestions that cancer patients there had experienced a reduction in pain because of Krebiozen.[49]

Ivy interpreted the committee's report entirely differently. "Once again premature and distorted publicity has misinformed the public about Krebiozen," he said. "Instead of finding Krebiozen ineffective, the Cole Committee Report has agreed with my previous conclusions, namely, that favorable changes occur with sufficient frequency after the administration of Krebiozen as to warrant further careful investigation." Ivy was not necessarily wrong. Warren Cole wrote to him privately that the committee's "findings and conclusions concerning the major issues were primarily a restatement of your conclusions." The committee had in fact recommended further investigation of the drug.[50]

Further investigation, though, was contingent on the Durovics sharing information that so far they had been unwilling to reveal. President Stoddard again met with the U of I Board of Trustees in late September. He recommended that Ivy get from the Durovics "all data, descriptions and formulations necessary to ascertain the chemical nature of Krebiozen and to undertake its biological preparation," with the understanding that the brothers' financial rights were to be fully protected. Stoddard also recommended the appointment of a new committee to be chaired by U of I physiology head Robert Johnson. It would be charged with analyzing samples of the drug, whereas the Cole Committee had been charged only with analyzing Ivy's case studies. "If for any reason the originators of Krebiozen cannot or will not cooperate effectively in carrying out this plan," said Stoddard, "I shall ask that there be no allowance of time, funds, space, equipment, patients or printing in behalf of any staff member of the University of Illinois for the clinical utilization of Krebiozen, and that every effort be made to dissociate Krebiozen from research or service programs." The trustees approved Stoddard's recommendations. "The next move is up to the Durovics," Park Livingston told the *Tribune*. "I hope they will see fit to accept the offer to be made by Dr. Stoddard to arrive at the solution of this problem in the American way." Stevan Durovic said that he and his brother would think about it; then he repeated that "certain powerful interests" were conspiring against them.[51]

At the end of September, medical dean Stanley Olson announced that he was leaving the U of I to take a similar position at Baylor University in Texas. In a statement to department heads in the College of Medicine, Olson said that Krebiozen had fatally compromised Ivy's effectiveness as an administrator. "This controversy has occupied and will continue to occupy a major share of the vice president's attention at a time when we have an unprecedented demand for leadership to prepare for the expansion which is about to take place," said Olson in referring to the U of I medical programs' ambitious development plans in Chicago. He added that "the basis for such leadership has been all but destroyed." Even though many faculty had lost confidence in Ivy, Olson had been limited in his ability to do anything about it, for Ivy as vice president was his administrative superior, and criticism of Ivy could have been seen as being motivated by personal ambition; some pro-Ivy people already suspected that Olson was angling for the vice president job. "I have assured myself that it is now unlikely that anything can or will be done to resolve these serious problems," said Olson in his statement. "I have been given an opportunity to employ my efforts elsewhere without an unreasonable handicap. The job here is tough enough at best—to do it under the present circumstances seems impossible." Olson shared a copy of his statement with President Stoddard, who told Provost Griffith that he had become profoundly concerned about the whole situation.[52]

In October, the *Chicago Herald-American* began running a series of articles on Krebiozen written by reporter Effie Alley. The Hearst-owned newspaper exceeded even the *Tribune* in its conservatism. It would run a front-page editorial that same month urging its readers to elect Dwight Eisenhower as president and Republicans to Congress "to rid the nation of the Socialism, corruption, fumbling and squandering that have saddled us with debt, curtailed our liberties, rifled our pockets and plunged us into a needless and never-ending war." Alley was a veteran science and medicine writer who later would become an antiabortion activist.[53]

Unlike the *Tribune*, the *Herald-American* adopted a pro-Krebiozen stance. Alley had obtained a copy of Ivy's report to the Cole Committee, and she interviewed several people with cancer who had received the drug and claimed that it had helped them, although Alley included little hard evidence in her stories to back those claims. A forty-seven-year-old Chicago woman related that her pain and her tumor had disappeared. "I can truthfully say I haven't had a sick day since I started taking Krebiozen," she said. "It's been a lot different with my friend. She had an operation for cancer about two years ago but the thing came back. Then she took X-ray [radiation treatment]. She's had a miserable time, constantly ailing. I think I'm lucky to have escaped that." Similar testimonials came from the family of Gary Cathcart in Wyoming (though Cathcart—like the other Krebiozen patients in Alley's stories—was not identified by name); from a woman in Wisconsin; from a doctor in Canada; and from several other people in the Chicago area. A fifty-year-old lawyer said that his doctor had told him that he probably had only a few months to live, with the doctor recommending radiation therapy. "I didn't go for that," the lawyer told Alley. He tried Krebiozen instead: "I'll never forget how I felt after they gave it to me. It was a real sense of triumph. . . . All I know is that I felt immensely better within three days. It could have been psychological, but I don't think so." The lawyer said that he already had lived twenty months longer than what his doctor had suggested was likely, which had allowed the man to return to work and make provisions for his family: "But of course, I hope for more—a normal span for myself and a great many other cancer victims. That's what it seems to me krebiozen promises."[54]

Ivy wrote to the *Herald-American* to register his "personal objection" to Alley's series and to other press reports about Krebiozen's apparent successes. He said that such stories could raise undue hopes in people with cancer while further alienating the medical establishment. "I cannot, however, deny the truth or validity of the articles now appearing in The Herald-American," Ivy was careful to add. "It is apparent that they are based on actual hospital records and case histories." He said that certain of his colleagues believed that he "sought to extend this scientific question to the newspapers instead of limiting it to the laboratory and the clinic where it properly should be confined. Anyone knowing me and my work and the procedures I have followed in the past should know that this is not the case."[55]

Meanwhile, Ivy was trying to persuade the Durovic brothers to comply with the U of I's requirements for continuing clinical tests of Krebiozen. For the past three years, he had urged them to reveal the secret of the drug's composition and preparation through a patent application. Now, Ivy made a circuitous effort to enlist President Stoddard into swaying the brothers. Ivy drafted a letter that he gave to Robert Johnson, who chaired the new U of I committee assigned to analyze Krebiozen. The letter was supposed to go to Stoddard for his signature and then be delivered to the Durovics. "In order that there will be no infringement of your technical, legal, or financial rights," the letter said, "Dr. Ivy has been instructed by me [Stoddard] to accept from you no descriptions, formulations, or technological procedures for the preparation of Krebiozen or for the determination of its chemical nature until you have protected yourself by revealing all such information in a patent application." Stoddard refused to have anything to do with the letter. He told Ivy that a patent could have been taken care of "months or years ago." As for the Durovics' rights, "neither the Johnson Committee nor any member of the staff of the University has the slightest interest in abridging such rights even though they would seem, from the conclusions of the Cole Committee, to possess no substantial value." Ivy and the Durovics were instructed to supply the Johnson Committee with three to four thousand ampules of the drug for analysis along with the complete chemical and manufacturing information no later than October 21.[56]

The Durovics seemed receptive at first, even though Stevan was still telling the newspapers of a conspiracy against them.[57] "We are eager to make available to the University of Illinois all information we possess regarding Krebiozen together with all the manufacturing details," Stevan wrote to Ivy. However, he and his brother needed the university to give them a clearer offer of protection, and they also needed more time, as the required information about the drug had to be translated from the Durovics' native tongue into English. The deadline was stretched into November. The Durovics then said that they still had not been given an adequate guarantee of their rights, and they still needed more time. "In order to be free to make complete disclosure we must in honor obtain the approval of other persons who are legitimately concerned regarding such protection, as we have prior obligations to these other persons which we cannot ignore," they told Ivy. It was extremely expensive to produce Krebiozen, they said; it took more than three thousand horses and cost more than $1.3 million to produce just two grams of the drug. There was no way that they could give the U of I three to four thousand ampules. They might possibly be able to provide thirty to forty milligrams of Krebiozen, but first a new batch would have to be produced. That process would have to happen in Argentina, and it would take six months, if not longer.[58]

Another article by Effie Alley appeared in the *Herald-American*. It quoted Stevan Durovic as saying that the U of I was making "unprecedented" demands for proprietary information: "The type of information now demanded could not be obtained even on so widely used a remedy as penicillin." The *Herald-American* claimed that it had confirmed the correctness of Durovic's stand through its checks with pharmaceutical companies. "That would be competitive information. Such things are never given out," Eli Lilly's vice president told the newspaper. The paper did not report that Eli Lilly had immediately withdrawn its financial offer to Durovic after he refused to share any details about the preparation of the drug, just as he was doing now with the U of I.[59]

Having concluded that it was futile to try to get the necessary information about Krebiozen from Ivy and the Durovics, the Johnson Committee asked to be discharged. President Stoddard granted that request on November 14. That same day, the president issued a report to the U of I Board of Trustees, which he simultaneously made public. He recapped his actions following the Cole Committee report, in particular his directive that if Krebiozen's originators did not cooperate with the U of I, the university would sever itself from the drug. Stoddard now declared that "there are to be no further clinical uses or determinations of Krebiozen on the part of staff members of the University of Illinois at any time" and that "Krebiozen henceforth is to be dissociated from research or service programs." He indicated that he was informing Ivy of those prohibitions.[60]

Had Stoddard simply stopped there in his report, it is conceivable that the entire Krebiozen saga might have turned out differently, with the controversy soon melting away. However, Stoddard did not stop there. He was angry. Northwestern University had speedily rejected Stevan Durovic and his medicine. Durovic then had gone to the U of I, whose vice president had proceeded to announce Krebiozen to the world without bothering to inform Stoddard or other top university officials in advance. It now had been more than a year since the AMA had said that Krebiozen was of no value in treating cancer, a verdict shared by *Science*, the *New England Journal of Medicine*, the National Research Council, the Institute of Medicine of Chicago, the Chicago Medical Society, the Champaign County Medical Society, and even the *Chicago Tribune*. U of I medical dean Stanley Olson had quit in disgust over the affair. He had disparaged the U of I's administration as being "almost mystical in character"; although Olson aimed that jibe at Ivy, he also was plainly mystified at Stoddard's refusal to act against Krebiozen.[61] For his part, Stoddard believed that he had given Ivy and the Durovics every opportunity—in truth, too many opportunities—to prove the drug's worth. He had appointed two separate committees to assist in that task. He had, in fact, sought to play the role of president-as-mediator in supporting Ivy and trying to placate other backers of the drug. The Durovics had responded by ignoring the U of I's requests for information and denigrating the university in the press, and Ivy seemed unable or unwilling to do anything about it. Enough was enough.

Consequently, Stoddard wrote in his report that he wished to "make a few final remarks." He said that the events surrounding Krebiozen had been "fantastic," in the sense of them being beyond belief. "The originators of the drug still speak of their need for 'protection,' as if the drug possessed value," wrote Stoddard. "Actually all the University of Illinois sought to do, following the report of the Cole Committee, was to solve the mystery of a preparation already discredited in medical practice." The Krebiozen affair had been "damaging to the scientific reputation of the University of Illinois. It is to be hoped that the present divorcement will have restorative value." Stoddard ended by saying that the Durovics' refusal to provide samples of the drug for analysis was especially telling: "it would appear that we really might have found nothing in the ampules and, therefore, could not be allowed to look for it. It is my considered opinion that, except possibly as a common, harmless, inexpensive ingredient, *Krebiozen does not exist*."[62]

In underlining those final four words, Stoddard likely believed that he had buried Krebiozen once and for all. Instead, he would give the mystery drug a jolt of new life while getting buried himself.

CHAPTER 3

Conspiracies and Circuses

Reaction to George Stoddard's anti-Krebiozen order was swift and fiercely divided, and it manifested itself in a manner typical of both government and academia: a torrent of meetings, memos, statements, resolutions, and reports. On November 21, 1952, one week after Stoddard's edict, the University of Illinois College of Medicine faculty met in Chicago to decide whether to endorse two statements forwarded by their executive committee—the first expressing regret about Andrew Ivy's role in promoting Krebiozen and the second supporting Stoddard's stand against the drug. The meeting turned into what one attendee described as "a knock-down-and-drag-out affair the like of which has never before been seen in the history of the institution." Ivy did not attend, but one of his allies read aloud a statement from him. Ivy reiterated his conviction that Krebiozen was "biologically active" in the cancer patient, supposedly consistent with the Cole Committee's tepid observation that the drug was not necessarily "devoid of biological activity." One medical professor introduced a resolution declaring that Stoddard's action against Krebiozen "might end for every one of us a tradition of freedom of research within a great university" while also endangering "the future of any new idea." The faculty defeated the resolution; and, after further angry debate, it voted to endorse both of the executive committee statements, albeit only narrowly when it came to supporting Stoddard's position. Afterward, medical dean Stanley Olson—who was about to leave the U of I for good—referred reporters' questions to Stoddard, saying that Krebiozen was now "the president's show."[1]

Stoddard already had heard from U of I trustee Frances Watkins. She wrote to the president that his anti-Krebiozen statement had been "bad for the University from a public relations standpoint; that it worsened the unhappy administrative situation in the [U of I's Chicago] professional schools; and that it was an unnecessary public personal blow at Dr. Ivy." She added that it would have been far preferable for Stoddard to say simply that the university was dissociating itself from Krebiozen and to wait to make any statement at all until after he had received the backing of the trustees at their scheduled November 28 meeting. Stoddard, who believed that he only had done what the trustees already had granted him the authority to do, wrote back to Watkins that the "administrative situation in the College of Medicine could hardly be worsened" and that the "only hope of saving any vestige of Ivy's professional status is to get him to repudiate the drug and the Durovics who have deceived him." In a letter to Illinois governor Adlai Stevenson, who would soon leave office after losing the US presidential election to Dwight Eisenhower, Stoddard was even more blunt: "It has become plain as daylight that Dr. Ivy has fallen under the evil influence of a pair of international adventurers. The only thing they have contributed to a drug which probably does not exist is a strong smell."[2]

Stoddard followed his initial edict against Krebiozen with an expanded report for the trustees to consider at their upcoming meeting. He said that Ivy's work on Krebiozen had violated the standard methods and safeguards of academic research, and thus the president had no choice but to prohibit further investigation of the drug at the university. "There is indeed a humane debt owed to persons in pain, who may include our own loved ones, but the debt can only be paid the hard way," Stoddard said. "To this hard way of rigorous research and testing the University of Illinois will continue to devote its best efforts." Saying that Ivy had lost the confidence of a majority of the Chicago professional colleges' faculty, Stoddard recommended that Ivy's vice president position be eliminated, with Ivy still heading the Department of Clinical Science and still being able to work on Krebiozen on his own time outside the university. The president further recommended that whoever would become the new College of Medicine dean also be made executive dean of all three professional colleges. That move would restore the arrangement that had been in place prior to Ivy's hiring. It reflected the reality that at least 85 percent of the three colleges' students and faculty resided in the medical college, with much smaller percentages in dentistry and pharmacy. Still, many dentistry and pharmacy faculty members believed that such a move would unfairly marginalize them. Abolishing Ivy's administrative post also would strike many of his supporters as further unwarranted humiliation.[3]

If Ivy voluntarily resigned the vice presidency, some of the tension might be defused. A number of Ivy's friends believed that he would in fact resign, with Ivy's own wife urging him to do so. U of I provost Coleman Griffith, who was considered to be Stoddard's right-hand man, also was a pioneering sports psychologist; during the late 1930s he had even provided his scholarly expertise to the Chicago Cubs baseball team, which had not been especially receptive to his input. Griffith now tried to use psychology on Ivy by writing to the vice president without Stoddard's knowledge. Griffith told Ivy that his resignation would "save the University of Illinois and all of its deeply interested friends and staff members from a head-on clash between two sets of ideas and opinions which, in and of themselves, have no yielding points." It also would enable Ivy to regain "the respect and admiration of those of your colleagues and friends in all fields of science all over the country who are bewildered and distressed by your recent activities."[4]

Griffith was no more successful with Ivy than he had been with the Cubs. Ivy had no intention of repudiating Krebiozen, at least not until after the drug had received the careful testing that he believed it deserved. He wrote in his own statement to the Board of Trustees that "if the results show that Krebiozen is *not* active in the cancer patient, which I believe is highly improbable," he would be the first to say so publicly. Stevan Durovic turned to *Chicago Herald-American* reporter Effie Alley to leak more details of Ivy's report to the Cole Committee. The report claimed that 70 percent of people with terminal cancer who had taken Krebiozen experienced benefits ranging from pain reduction to complete remission of their disease.[5]

As for Ivy resigning the vice presidency, highly placed friends argued against it. Some U of I trustees besides Frances Watkins were unhappy with President Stoddard. One unnamed trustee told the press that if the president could shut down a faculty member's research, he could also tell the faculty member "what church to go to, what to teach, [and] even what friends he might have." State lawmakers were lambasting Stoddard as well. Republican WB Westbrook of Harrisburg in southern Illinois called the president's Krebiozen edict an "administrative blunder." Chicago Republican Charles Jenkins said that Stoddard was "dictatorial" and noted that Ivy had been personally responsible for helping the university get bigger appropriations from the legislature. Most critical of all was Chicago Democrat Roland Libonati. "If Doctor Ivy is forced out of the university in a summary manner, we'll investigate the whole set-up at the university," Libonati said, adding that the university's "policy toward research should be determined by the trustees who are elected by the people—not by President Stoddard." Libonati and Jenkins joined fellow Chicago legislators Peter J. Miller and Vito Marzullo in demanding that the trustees keep Ivy from resigning.[6]

The November 28 U of I Board of Trustees meeting in Chicago drew unprecedented media attention, including what was said to be the first-ever appearance of television cameras at a trustee meeting. The attendees included lawyers, state lawmakers, U of I medical professors, a Roman Catholic priest, and two women with cancer who said that Krebiozen had saved their lives. At the meeting's scheduled start time, President Stoddard and Provost Griffith were seated at their usual places, but no trustees were present; they were huddling in a separate room, and Ivy was rumored to be with them. The meeting finally began twenty-five minutes late with Ivy in attendance. Stoddard recited his report explaining his actions against Krebiozen and recommending the elimination of Ivy's vice presidency. The trustees voted unanimously to refer Stoddard's recommendations to a committee. After the meeting adjourned, the Krebiozen Research Foundation accused Stoddard of employing "Hitler's 'big lie' technique," and Libonati told reporters that "most of the legislators are questioning the retention of Stoddard as president of the university."[7]

In actuality, some legislators were more positively disposed toward Stoddard, at least to the extent of trying to temper the fury surrounding Krebiozen. A legislative commission that visited the U of I's Chicago facilities commended the "integrity and courage" of both Stoddard and Ivy. If lawmakers differed in their attitudes toward the controversy, so too did the news media. The Champaign *News-Gazette* continued giving voice to such anti-Stoddard partisans as Libonati, while the *Chicago Herald-American* kept printing Alley's pro-Krebiozen articles. She highlighted unpublished portions of the Cole Committee report that allegedly showed how Krebiozen benefited cancer patients, the implication being that the university had deliberately suppressed those parts of the report.[8] Meanwhile, the *Daily Illini* student newspaper—after first sharply questioning Stoddard's actions—decried growing legislative meddling in the Krebiozen affair. The *Chicago Daily News* said that Ivy "should relieve the university of its present embarrassing association with Krebiozen," although the paper stopped short of calling for his resignation. And the *Chicago Tribune*, which regularly published anti-Krebiozen editorials, blasted Ivy and the Durovics for using a secret remedy: "No physician is justified in subjecting a patient to treatment under such conditions."[9]

Stoddard enjoyed robust support from the health-care community. The Chicago Medical Society passed a resolution supporting his anti-Krebiozen order, and the executive committee of the U of I College of Medicine declared that "Dr. Ivy has acted in an unfortunate, unscientific, and unethical manner in dealing with 'Krebiozen'."[10] A U of I faculty senate committee headed by chemistry professor Roger Adams agreed with Stoddard that "the failure to employ proper scientific procedures and precautions in the research on Krebiozen is evidence of neglect of established scientific principles." Adams had received a note from Ivy's mentor, Anton J. Carlson, saying that adherence to scientific principles was especially important in cancer's case because the disease attracted so much quackery. In addition, Adams's committee, along with another faculty senate committee, found no infringement of Ivy's academic freedom. According to the American Association of University Professors, although professors were "entitled to full freedom in research and in the publication of the results," they also were obligated to adhere to "a scholar's method" and "a scholar's spirit," and it was up to fellow faculty members to determine whether that method and spirit had been abused. Ivy's academic peers judged that he had flouted scholarly standards, and therefore he could not legitimately claim that his academic freedom had been violated.[11]

Just prior to the next Board of Trustees meeting on December 22, the U of I faculty senate passed a new resolution. It asked the trustees "to protect the Faculty in the pursuit of its educational and scientific aims from undue influence or interference." The senate had reason to be concerned, as the December trustees meeting outdid the previous month's meeting in its tumult. Ignoring Stoddard's recommendation to eliminate Ivy's vice presidency, the board instead granted Ivy a six-month leave without pay to continue his research on Krebiozen. Then came yet another new resolution, which triggered an uproar. It was proposed by trustee Vernon Nickell, and it lavished praise on Ivy, including praise for his administration of the Chicago professional colleges. A fellow trustee denounced Nickell for springing the matter on the board with no warning. When the board voted to refer the resolution to a committee, Roland Libonati seized the floor. "I don't think the board used good sense in sending this to a committee. We don't like it," he shouted. There were raucous cheers from Ivy's supporters amid popping flashbulbs from news photographers. Fellow state lawmaker Charles Jenkins told the board that Ivy was being "crucified like Jesus Christ." The trustees then told Nickell to redraft his resolution with the understanding that it likely would pass the next time that they met, while Libonati said that he would call for a legislative committee to investigate the university.[12]

Ivy refused to make a statement at the board meeting, despite impassioned pleas from Libonati and other attendees that he do so. Otherwise, Ivy was hardly keeping quiet. He said that freedom of research "should not be forgotten in the United States although it is forgotten under totalitarian government." He castigated the College of Medicine executive committee for "intemperance and angry emotionalism," and he denied that he was giving false hope to people with cancer: "I am perfectly willing to let this whole matter turn upon the question of hope vs. suspicion, and to cast my lot with the former. Certainly I never want my soul to be so dead that I am hopeless myself or seek to make others hopeless." Regarding assertions that the doctors administering Krebiozen had no expertise in oncology, Ivy said that "the general practitioner is just as competent as the 'cancer expert'" in evaluating patients. As for criticisms of Krebiozen being quackery, Ivy declared that "like my forefathers who pioneered in our country since the 1620s, the greater the harassment, the greater the threats, the greater the breaches of fair play, the greater becomes my determination to set up and supervise the conduct of a strictly controlled study" of the drug.[13]

Ivy was notoriously stubborn. He liked to tell the story of being a child in turn-of-the-century Cape Girardeau, Missouri, and being cornered by an angry goat. Ivy charged headfirst at the goat and scared it away. Even after becoming a distinguished physiologist, he still called himself a "hillbilly and swamp angel." A "swamp angel" was a cannon that had been used in the US Civil War. The implication was clear: Ivy was no effete big-city intellectual who handed down edicts. He was a small-town, hard-working man of the people, and he was not to be trifled with.[14]

Although Ivy surely did not know it, while he was a child, "swamp angel" was also the name of a patent medicine. It was claimed to cure tumors, goiters, tuberculosis, asthma, diarrhea, colic, rheumatism, deafness, baldness, dandruff, and ailments of the kidney, bladder, and liver. "Pour out thirty drops of Swamp Angel Medicine in sugar and swallow it, close your mouth, and you can feel liquid fire and gases coming through every air-cell of your lungs and passing off through the nostrils," advertisements proclaimed, adding that Swamp Angel Medicine also killed spiders and flies. The advertisements included a banner headline: "BELIEVE AND LIVE, DISBELIEVE AND YOU MAY DIE."[15]

More than half a century later, Krebiozen was posing its own choice between belief and disbelief. Was it just another phony patent medicine formulated for a new generation of suckers? Or was it the outstanding miracle drug of its time, saved from oblivion by an intrepid doctor who refused to be cowed?

• • •

Noxious concoctions like Swamp Angel Medicine had helped prompt the US government to enact the Pure Food and Drug Act in 1906 and the American Medical Association to ramp up its war against quackery. Yet quackery did not disappear. Its practitioners became more sophisticated in employing new media technologies and in turning the AMA into a handy foil. In the 1920s, John Brinkley used his Kansas radio station to extoll his goat-gland transplant therapy and brand the AMA as "the Amalgamated Meatcutters Association." After losing both his radio license and medical license in 1930, Brinkley unsuccessfully ran for Kansas governor before moving to Texas and starting a new radio station just across the border in Mexico. Norman Baker of Muscatine, Iowa, similarly used radio in the 1920s and 1930s to promote a quack cancer drug and attack representatives of organized medicine. "Their only concern for the poor cancer patient is to get his money, and fulfill the definition of the initials, M.D., meaning 'more dough,'" said Baker. He likened the AMA to an octopus whose arms extended "into every home, into every school, into every college, into every living breathing soul in America." He even sued the AMA for libel but lost.[16]

In the years just before Krebiozen's emergence, William Frederick Koch and Harry Hoxsey were both frequently in the news. Koch's purported cancer cure was first said to be derived from cow brains and hearts; it then was said to be a synthetic antitoxin that restored natural immunity to cancer, and it was given a scientific-sounding name: Glyoxylide. Koch, who held not only an MD but also a PhD from the University of Michigan, used his credentials to bolster his credibility. The Food and Drug Administration twice launched criminal prosecutions of him in the 1940s, using Anton Carlson as an expert witness. Both times, the FDA lost, as unanimous jury verdicts against Koch proved impossible. Koch eventually moved his operations to Brazil. In his stead, Hoxsey became the most prominent proponent of nonstandard cancer treatment in the US with his Hoxsey Therapy administered to thousands of patients in his Dallas, Texas, clinic. Hoxsey—who first launched his career in Illinois and who also briefly allied himself with Norman Baker—successfully sued both the Hearst newspaper chain and the AMA's Morris Fishbein for their criticisms of him, although he received only token cash awards. He won support from US senators and a right-wing journalist who became his publicist. "Hitler, Mussolini, and Stalin—all put together—never had as much dictatorial power as is possessed by the licensed medical men of these free United States," Hoxsey said. The FDA won an injunction against him in 1951, which he fiercely resisted.[17]

Andrew Ivy was no friend of Hoxsey. Ivy had even helped investigate Hoxsey's Texas clinic for the American Cancer Society in 1949, and he had reported that Hoxsey's claimed cancer cures were people who never had the disease to begin with or else had been cured by mainstream medicine. Significantly, though, Ivy also would argue that Hoxsey's therapy should receive an impartial scientific test instead of being summarily rejected by the likes of the AMA. As Ivy put it, "the way the A.M.A. and organized groups now operate tends to produce public support of alleged 'quacks' and 'quack remedies.'" With Ivy presently linked to Krebiozen, he and his allies would follow the script established by Brinkley, Baker, Koch, and Hoxsey. The AMA became the enemy, with its treasurer JJ Moore supposedly having conspired with Ed Moore and Kenneth Brainard to grab control of the drug or else crush it through a trumped-up AMA report denying its value. It helped, of course, that the AMA was already deeply unpopular among many people for its antagonism toward group health insurance and other health-care reforms.[18]

Ivy also would follow Koch's example in assuming the role of a distinguished scientist who was being persecuted for daring to question conventional wisdom: the so-called "Galileo ploy," which, in Ivy's case, might have been more appropriately called "the Pasteur ploy." The 1936 Hollywood movie *The Story of Louis Pasteur* had starred Paul Muni as the courageous doctor who overcame widespread scorn from the medical establishment in winning scientific acceptance of his theory that microbes caused disease. (The 1940 film *Dr. Ehrlich's Magic Bullet*, starring Edward G. Robinson as Paul Ehrlich, had similarly celebrated the heroic maverick scientist.) There even was a statue of Pasteur near Ivy's U of I office in Chicago. It bore a plaque with Pasteur's words: "One doesn't ask of one who suffers: what is your country and what is your religion? One merely says, you suffer. That is enough for me. You belong to me and I shall help you." Ivy likewise saw himself as upholding his moral responsibility to help people with cancer even in the face of misguided if not downright venal opposition.[19]

Ivy's stance resonated with legislative allies. US senator Paul Douglas had known Ivy for years, and the senator was sympathetic toward what he viewed as principled challenges to entrenched authority. Charles Jenkins, an African American Illinois state representative and civil-rights advocate, said that he held a "violent" interest in giving Krebiozen a fair chance after his wife's death from cancer.[20] Other state lawmakers from Chicago had extra motivation to defend Ivy. Peter J. Miller had battled the U of I and President Stoddard over the building contract for a new women's residence hall in Urbana; the contract had gone to one of Miller's Chicago friends whom the university had accused of cost overruns. The U of I eventually won the dispute with Miller, who told reporters that Stoddard had insulted him just by the way that the U of I president had looked at him.[21] Vito Marzullo had previously led an investigation of the U of I's medical programs. Having left school after the fourth grade, Marzullo was fond of denigrating college professors and intellectuals, which would not stop him from accepting an invitation to lecture on politics to a rapt audience at Harvard University.[22]

Ivy's biggest champion, Roland Libonati, was a seasoned practitioner of Chicago city politics. He said that he wore out his hat every three or four weeks by constantly doffing it to his constituents on the street. Libonati insisted that Ivy and the Durovic brothers needed protection against people like Stoddard. "The university is not a place for carpetbaggers," he said of Stoddard, who had come from the East. "No one person should have too much authority in the reappointment of deans and all that. Why should that be in the hands of the president?" Libonati said that he saw the U of I as "a public institution rather than belonging to the faculty alone," and he added that instead of trusting the judgment of university administrators, he preferred people "who are not too expert, who can see the general picture."[23]

Libonati and Marzullo were members of what was called the West Side bloc in the Illinois legislature. Miller also was said to be a member, although he would deny being one. The bloc was a bipartisan group of lawmakers from Chicago's West Side who regularly voted against anticrime measures; Libonati had been friends with Al Capone, and he used his law practice to defend other organized crime figures in court. The U of I's professional colleges and medical facilities were located in the West Side enclave known as Little Italy. One medical professor compared the neighborhood to "a southern Italian or Sicilian village" of small restaurants, shops, and "older two- and three-flat apartment buildings in varying states of repair and disrepair," some of which Libonati owned amid accusations that he was delinquent in upkeep and in property tax payments. The medical professor remembered that neighborhood residents treated U of I staff with indulgence: "Mugging or strong-arming of medical personnel was unheard of."[24]

In return, the neighborhood's political representatives expected the sort of patronage that had long been rampant in Chicago: a city that, according to newspaper columnist Mike Royko, could just as well change its slogan from *Urbs in Horto* ("City in a Garden") to *Ubi Est Mea* ("Where's Mine?"). Building contracts such as the one for the U of I residence hall went to well-connected friends, as did choice political jobs. Marzullo boasted of filling positions ranging from an assistant state's attorney and an assistant attorney general to electrical inspectors, street inspectors, and highway inspectors. It seemed that he also had expected to fill positions in the U of I's clinics and medical programs, especially because the university represented the largest public payroll in the area. When Marzullo's expectations were not met, he called legislative hearings in 1949, and medical dean John Youmans resigned soon afterward.[25]

It was now rumored—though not proved—that Ivy as U of I vice president was facilitating patronage through the expansion of the university's medical facilities in Chicago. For Provost Griffith, those rumors were another reason to eliminate Ivy's vice president position; Griffith believed that elected officials (including the West Side bloc, onetime state's attorney John Boyle, and U of I Board of Trustees president Park Livingston) were protecting Ivy in order to preserve the patronage that Ivy enabled through his administrative post. For his part, Ivy proudly touted the new funding and construction that he had helped bring to the university on the West Side, and he denied any underhandedness. The charges and countercharges only added to the acrimony surrounding Krebiozen and the new legislative hearings that would soon begin.[26]

• • •

The Illinois House executive committee approved the hearings in February 1953 at Libonati's behest. He claimed that because President Stoddard had "assumed powers which were not his" and had become a "puppet" of the individuals conspiring against Krebiozen, hearings were needed to investigate the alleged conspiracy and whatever role the U of I may have played in it. When Stoddard did not appear as invited before the executive committee, lawmakers tore into him, with one of them vowing to subpoena him. Andrew Ivy also did not appear before the committee, but John Boyle spoke on his behalf. Boyle had lost his state's attorney position after Cook County Democrats dropped him from their 1952 ticket for his missteps on the job. The *Chicago Daily News* had compared him to "a gent who shot championship pool—when nobody else was in the pool hall. But when somebody was watching, he missed most shots and even tore the felt on a few." Boyle subsequently had become Ivy's lawyer, and he sneeringly told state lawmakers that "many little men are saying they know more about medical ethics than Dr. Ivy." Clearly, Stoddard was deemed to be chief among those "little men." The state's new Republican governor, William Stratton, also was at odds with the university president. According to one legislator, there was no hope of rapprochement between Stratton and Stoddard: "It's impossible. They don't even eat the same kind of food."[27]

Some Republican state lawmakers had misgivings about the Krebiozen hearings. Everett Peters, from the central Illinois town of St. Joseph, called the people pushing for the hearings "fanatics." Elbert Smith of Decatur said that the U of I "must be recognized as having power to determine the subjects on which it is to engage in research," and he added that the hearings would unfairly undermine confidence in the university's trustees. Robert McClory, who represented the Chicago suburb of Lake Bluff, said that the U of I's medical staff would "see great harm to the research hospital and the university in such an inquisition." Yet the legislature as a whole voted to go ahead with the hearings. They would be overseen by a bipartisan committee of fourteen lawmakers, including Libonati. Chicago Republican William Pollack reluctantly agreed to serve as chair. The stated goal was to keep the proceedings from turning into a "circus."[28]

When the hearings began in Springfield in March, it quickly became apparent that not only had the circus arrived, but also that it was prepared for a lengthy run. Chicago attorney John Sembower, who was serving as Ivy's legal counsel along with Boyle, announced that affidavits would show how the AMA had joined the dastardly plot against Krebiozen and how the conspiracy reached all the way to South America. Ivy and Stoddard both testified under oath, with Ivy calling for a fair test to prove or disprove Krebiozen's value in treating cancer. He heatedly told "petty critics" to "keep their mouths shut and their pens dry until the only worthy question is answered with finality." Stoddard, in turn, questioned everything about the drug: "What *is* Krebiozen? How is it produced? What standard tests have been applied to it? Has it ever been used for the treatment of diseases other than malignant tumors? If, as the Durovics claim, a batch of Krebiozen in paraffin solution was spoiled by improper testing methods, why was none subsequently made available by *good* testing methods?" Stoddard's questions were left hanging as the hearings adjourned until April. They would move to the Chicago city council chambers, and television and radio coverage would be welcomed.[29]

In the interim, Stoddard sent a new report to the Krebiozen legislative committee under the heading, "The Key to the Puzzle—the Durovics." The U of I was trying to uncover information about the brothers' past. Some biographical details that the Durovics had given to the press turned out to be true. Stevan did hold a Yugoslavian medical degree, and he did offer his services to the US Army in 1942; the army had turned him down with thanks for his "patriotic offer." Marko really had been connected to a Yugoslavian munitions company called Vistad.[30] Other information, though, raised suspicions. There was no record of Stevan having published any research. (When questioned about this, Stevan had a simple retort: "I was working, not writing.") A U of I professor who visited the Durovics' former headquarters in Argentina found only primitive laboratory facilities and no one with any knowledge of Krebiozen, which was supposed to have originated there. A *Chicago Tribune* correspondent in Latin America, Jules Dubois, similarly found no evidence that Krebiozen ever had been produced in Argentina; he agreed with Stoddard that "Krebiozen might be a Durovic myth."[31]

The university also received a letter from an Argentinian doctor saying that Stevan had used his Kositerin hypertension medicine to ingratiate himself with high officials in Juan Perón's government. The Perón regime had tried to boost national pride and the Argentinian economy through supposed miracle drugs and inventions. In 1951, the regime announced that it had built a revolutionary fusion power device called a Thermotron that had been invented by a mysterious European expatriate not unlike Stevan. The device turned out to be useless.[32] Stevan even had administered Kositerin to a prominent Argentinian aviator whose hypertension had been unaffected and who had dropped dead soon afterward. "I think Durovic is a very dangerous bird," the letter writer said. President Stoddard therefore urged the legislative committee to investigate the two brothers, particularly Stevan, whom Stoddard called "a living question mark."[33]

The *Champaign-Urbana Courier* and its editor, Robert Sink, had been digging into the Durovics' checkered record as well. Under Sink, the *Courier* had taken a more sympathetic stance toward Stoddard's presidency than had its competitor, the *News-Gazette*. The paper reported Anton Carlson's comments that "the probability that a single individual within the space of a few years has discovered two miracle drugs, one a specific for cancer and the other for hypertension, seems extremely unlikely." Carlson opined that Krebiozen was actually Kositerin under a different label. Sink also spoke with Northwestern University president J. Roscoe Miller, who recalled Northwestern's negative experiences with Durovic and Kositerin and who added that Durovic never had mentioned Krebiozen. Sink asked in the *Courier* whether Durovic's idea for Krebiozen had been "born in a taxi" ferrying the Yugoslavian doctor from Northwestern to Ivy's office at the U of I. In addition, Sink wrote a column titled "Parable of the Potent Potion" that satirized the Durovics and Andrew Ivy, whom Sink branded as "Dr. Simon Pure."[34]

Notwithstanding, the *Courier* piled attention on the Krebiozen hearings and saw its circulation increase. Other news media also avidly followed the hearings, including the *Chicago Tribune*, even though that newspaper called the legislative committee "a group whose judgment of the merits of a horse liniment wouldn't be accepted seriously." One journalist observed in the *Saturday Evening Post* that the proceedings, which were conducted under blinding television lights and flashbulbs, featured "surely some of the most uproarious and fantastic testimony ever given in a legislative body. . . . Witnesses testified in several languages, often loudly. Somebody seemed always to be just getting off a boat or airplane to argue with the committee. [Roland] Libonati and other committee members kept jumping up and making angry speeches. Chairman William E. Pollack once said sadly, 'I don't know what I'm doing here—the committee doesn't pay any attention to me.'"[35]

The conspiracy charges dominated the hearings. Peter Neskow testified that AMA treasurer JJ Moore had told the Durovics to give Krebiozen's distribution rights to Ed Moore and Kenneth Brainard. The Durovics' attorney, Nick Stepanovich, who had befriended the brothers and helped

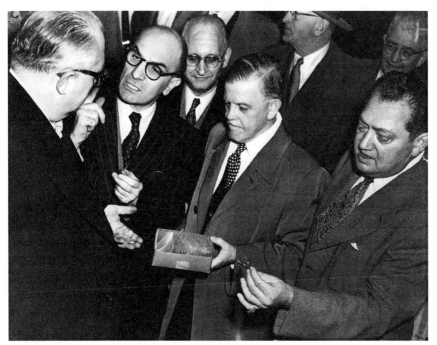

A typically tumultuous moment during the 1953 Illinois legislative committee hearings on Krebiozen. Committee chair William Pollack (far left) listens to an animated Stevan Durovic (second from left). Attorney Randolph Bohrer (far right) interjects while skeptically examining Krebiozen ampules from a box held by Andrew Ivy (second from right). (Chicago Tribune/TCA)

get them permanent residency in the United States, also testified on their behalf. (Only three months earlier, the Durovics had surreptitiously tried to dump Stepanovich as their lawyer while threatening to move to a new country where they could make money from Krebiozen.) Stepanovich read testimonials for Krebiozen from US senator Arthur Vandenberg's doctor and from Wallace Graham, a onetime White House physician who had given the drug to members of the US Army. In addition, Stepanovich disclosed Eli Lilly's million-dollar offer for the drug. The disclosure was intended to counter Stoddard's charges that Krebiozen did not exist: how could a nonexistent medicine command such a price? It also was intended to bolster claims of a conspiracy against Krebiozen, with so much money at stake.[36]

Argentinian commodore Alberto Barriera and his secretary, Ana Dorotea Schmidt, made an especially dramatic appearance. Barriera testified that he had pretended to be the Durovics' enemy, whereas in reality he was trying to document JJ Moore's plot to seize control of the drug. Barriera and Schmidt had even secretly recorded their phone conversations with Moore. The recordings were played for the legislative committee, but they revealed little other than Moore's animosity toward the Durovics. When Moore demanded to give his side of the story to the committee, he was told that he would have to wait. Instead, he held an impromptu news conference to deny the charges against him and call Krebiozen "one of the biggest fakes in cancer therapy in the last ten years."[37]

Accusation piled on accusation. A Roman Catholic priest claimed that Kenneth Brainard had implicitly threatened to kidnap Marko Durovic's son. Ivy charged that the AMA and Chicago cancer specialist Henry Szujewski had deliberately published "false and misleading" reports on Krebiozen. (A few months after the AMA's negative report on the drug in October 1951, Szujewski had issued his own negative assessment in the *Journal of the American Medical Association*.) Franklin Bing's letter warning Ivy that the AMA would ruin him was made public in a strategically edited form that made the letter sound like a threat. Bing's expressions of respect and affection for Ivy were omitted, as were Bing's observations in a separate letter that Ivy was associating with the wrong kind of people. Effie Alley of the *Chicago Herald-American* testified that an unnamed U of I faculty member had said that "Dr. Ivy has to go, but his stature is such that it will take a little while to destroy him." When a U of I attorney protested Alley's refusal to identify the faculty member, Alley's husband—an attorney himself—defended her right to protect a confidential source.[38]

There was pathos during the hearings when several Krebiozen patients were silently paraded through the meeting room. Ivy created fresh spectacle by displaying a tiny vial of Krebiozen powder to the legislative committee, again implicitly rebutting Stoddard's denial of the drug's existence. Stevan Durovic raised a ruckus of his own by momentarily vanishing from the hearing room and failing to testify as anticipated. After Durovic did take the stand, the proceedings slowed dramatically because of the constant translations from one language to another and the witness's recalcitrance. An AMA attorney managed to extract Durovic's admission that he had refused to divulge Krebiozen's formula to Eli Lilly, despite the company's million-dollar offer to him. Randolph Bohrer, the flamboyant attorney representing Ed Moore and Kenneth Brainard, indicated that he possessed incriminating documents against the Durovics. By now, though, it was May, and the Illinois legislative session was almost over. Further Krebiozen hearings were postponed until the fall.[39]

U of I president Stoddard had not been asked to provide additional testimony, and he joked that he could not remember the last time that he had remained quiet for so long. The U of I College of Medicine faculty, which had been sharply split on Stoddard a few months earlier, now voted overwhelmingly to express its full confidence in him.[40] However, powerful people did not share that confidence, and, through some conspiring of their own, they finally would bring Stoddard's presidency to an unceremonious end.

• • •

If Krebiozen was the biggest controversy surrounding Stoddard and the university, it was hardly the only one. Turmoil in the College of Commerce had not subsided with Dean Howard Bowen's forced resignation in December 1950. "As long as conditions exist where a member of the faculty goes down a hall opening doors and telling his colleagues that he is no longer on speaking terms with them, the situation is bad," one professor said. More faculty committees held more meetings and issued more reports to try to fix the situation, without much success. Many of Bowen's hires were leaving the university, and some professors were determined not to leave quietly. One departee issued a public statement that "freedom of teaching and research in my field" at the U of I "is no longer possible in terms of outside pressures—business, political, and journalistic—that have been brought to bear." Pressures also were brought to bear in the selection of a new U of I agriculture dean, as Illinois farming leaders and university benefactors pressured an out-of-state candidate for the position to withdraw.[41]

The U of I's broadcasting service, WILL, stirred anger on two fronts. Quincy Howe, formerly of CBS, had become a visiting professor of journalism at the university while delivering commentary on WILL radio. One Chicago attorney complained that Illinois taxpayers should not be forced to underwrite "a globalistic, Democratic propagandist." A more serious and protracted controversy developed over the university's efforts to start a television service. The Illinois Broadcasters Association charged that such a service would be "socialistic" and could harbor subversives. Then the U of I campus at Chicago's Navy Pier erupted in anger. The campus wanted to expand its curriculum from two years to four years, which President Stoddard opposed. A group of faculty issued a "declaration of independence" asserting that "the latest betrayal of the taxpayers of Illinois by Pres. George D. Stoddard and his trustee puppets leave secession as the only alternative."[42]

Illinois politicians continued taking potshots at the Stoddard administration. Republican state lawmaker Reed Cutler said that he was "ashamed" of the U of I and would remain so "until they get rid of that crew over there." Fellow Republican William Horsley said that he was "sick and tired of the pinkos" at the university, and he claimed that professors there were giving his son lower grades in retaliation for Horsley's support of antisubversion legislation. (The *Champaign-Urbana Courier* noted that Horsley's son had been on academic probation ever since he first enrolled at the university.) State auditor Orville Hodge pointed to the U of I's "poor public relations" as a rationale for auditing the university's books. Democrat Vito Marzullo introduced an anti-Stoddard, pro-Ivy bill requiring the university to maintain a vice president in charge of the Chicago professional colleges and allowing the trustees to fill that position without any input from the president.[43]

In June 1953, Stoddard delivered a speech titled "Paranoids versus the People" that received wide publicity. "It is alarmingly easy to poison the springs of public trust and confidence," Stoddard said. "In the United States of the mid-century, hate has been incorporated; it is a campaign." The U of I president charged that the campaign was being led by paranoid persons with delusions of grandeur and persecution. "The paranoid is always with us, but he prospers only in a sick world," Stoddard said in conclusion. "Reform him, cure him, confine him if you must, but under no circumstance believe him, imitate him, or give him power, for he will bring ruin."[44]

Harold "Red" Grange was no paranoid, nor was he especially political. He would forever be known as the legendary "Galloping Ghost" who had scored four touchdowns in twelve minutes for the Fighting Illini football team in a 1924 game. When he was offered big money to play professional football, Grange left the U of I without graduating. He later became a sports broadcaster. In 1950—during an upswing of the kind of anticommunist paranoia that Stoddard decried—Illinois Republicans had tapped Grange for their slate of candidates for the U of I Board of Trustees, replacing a Stoddard backer. Grange was elected easily despite refusing to campaign for the position. "I don't want any truck with pinks," he told reporters after his election, but he added that he had no knowledge of any "pinks" being on the faculty. His top priority as trustee seemed to be building a bigger basketball arena, while also opposing the university's purchases of abstract art and new pianos for the music school.[45]

According to his later recollection, Grange disliked being on the board: "I hadn't been a trustee more than a couple of days, and I started getting phone calls from politicians, telling me to put this guy or that guy to work or else you won't get your budget through. I don't believe it's the right way to run a university." Be that as it may, during a marathon board meeting late in the evening of July 24, 1953, Grange called for a trustees-only conference, and President Stoddard and Provost Griffith were asked to leave the room. At about midnight, the board called in Stoddard. "Prepare yourself for a shock," one of the trustees told him. Board president Park Livingston informed Stoddard that the trustees had voted six to three that they had no confidence in his presidency, with Grange having called for the vote. The president immediately scribbled and signed a letter of resignation. Griffith was then informed that the board also had voted no confidence in him and that he was being relieved of his administrative post. Longtime U of I comptroller Lloyd Morey was named acting president. In a separate move, the board removed Ivy as vice president, while keeping the vice president position intact and allowing Ivy to remain on the medical faculty.[46]

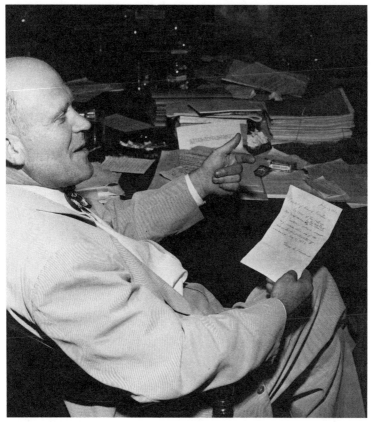

Park Livingston, president of the University of Illinois Board of Trustees, displays George Stoddard's hastily scribbled resignation note in July 1953. Livingston helped orchestrate Stoddard's ouster as U of I president. (Courtesy of the University of Illinois at Urbana-Champaign Archives, image 0011528)

The trustee was right to advise Stoddard to ready himself for a jolt, for both the U of I president and the provost had been oblivious of what was about to befall them; witnesses said that Stoddard appeared "dumbfounded" and Griffith turned "white as flour" when they heard the news. The three trustees who had voted to support Stoddard also had received no advance notice of their colleagues' plan to oust the administrators. But many other people had known what was coming. Governor Stratton was aware, as were Illinois labor leaders who had been unhappy that Stoddard permitted layoffs of some university workers in response to state budget cuts. Select journalists also had been tipped off. Even custodial staff at Urbana's Illini Union, where the trustees had met, knew that the firings were imminent. One custodian offered a bet of twenty-five dollars that Stoddard would be terminated, only to receive no takers.[47]

It was obvious that the firings had been carefully orchestrated and that Stratton and Livingston had played key roles. Livingston had lost to Stratton in the 1952 Illinois Republican gubernatorial primary, and news analysts speculated that Stoddard's dismissal could benefit both men politically: it might boost Livingston's popularity among Republicans and help him launch a US Senate bid, while also removing him as a potential future competitor to Stratton as governor. Livingston told the *Chicago Tribune* that trustees had grown dissatisfied with Stoddard over all the controversies surrounding his presidency. Among them were Stoddard's 1945 tussle with a Roman Catholic bishop over supposed godlessness; Stoddard's absences from the U of I to work for UNESCO; the protracted squabbles in the College of Commerce, the School of Music, and other academic units; and the constant charges of leftism at the university.[48]

Stoddard held no doubt about what really had sparked the no-confidence vote. "Krebiozen is to all this as slavery was to the war between the states," he told reporters. "There were other factors, but it needed a trigger." Stoddard also squarely blamed Livingston for his forced resignation, saying that the board president was the type of person who "exploits and debases the whole university idea to political needs in order to achieve political ambition." Stoddard said that Grange was "just a creature of Livingston's." In addition, Stoddard issued a lengthy public statement systematically defending what his administration had done about the controversies listed in the *Tribune*. Noting that many people wished for "a period of peace for the University of Illinois," Stoddard warned that "there could be a peace of the graveyard."[49]

There was little peace on campus in the immediate aftermath of Stoddard's ouster, even though it was summer and many students and faculty were absent. Eighteen academic department heads issued a joint letter condemning the firing, and a sociology professor quit the faculty to protest the trustees' actions. Nearly a thousand people marched to the president's house to give Stoddard a scroll pointedly expressing the campus's confidence in him. Wayne Johnston—one of the three pro-Stoddard trustees who had been deliberately left unaware about the planned no-confidence vote—excoriated the president's forced resignation, and for a time he threatened to resign himself. A large group of former U of I trustees and the executive committee of the university alumni association also registered their disapproval.[50] Although the Champaign *News-Gazette* predictably was pleased with Stoddard's departure, other newspapers blasted the "highhanded politicking," "bad motives and false issues," and "dirty political intrigue" underlying the firing. The *Daily Illini* student paper said that Stoddard had been "completely out of place in the choking atmosphere of conservatism and bigotry in the community, the legislature, and the state as a whole." Almost lost amid the rancor was the fact that Ivy also had lost his administrative position, much as Stoddard had recommended.[51]

The *Champaign-Urbana Courier*, while acknowledging Stoddard's occasional imperiousness and bursts of temper, concurred with the deposed president that Krebiozen had triggered his firing. "It is not too surprising that [Krebiozen] has attracted its sympathetic following," the paper editorialized. "The American public enjoys a good medicine show, just as it always enjoyed seeing W. C. Fields trim the suckers. It knows the snake oil won't help grandma's rheumatism, but it's soothing, for a while, to be fooled." For the same reason, people felt compelled "to throw out the academic spoilsport who says that the snake oil is no good." The real test now, said the *Courier*, was whether U of I trustees (and, presumably, Illinois lawmakers) would finally display "the courage to embrace the truth when rascality is more fun."[52]

• • •

The medicine show-cum-circus of the Illinois Krebiozen hearings still had a while to run, with the hearings resuming in Chicago in September. Ivy and Stevan Durovic spent substantial time being cross-examined by attorneys for the AMA and by Randolph Bohrer, the attorney for Ed Moore and Kenneth Brainard. It was revealed that Ivy did not know whether Krebiozen and Kositerin were the same drug, did not know of reports that Krebiozen was being sold in Uruguay, and did not know that John Pickering, who had issued the exaggerated claims for Krebiozen before Ivy's Drake Hotel presentation, had worked for John Boyle. But Ivy rejected suggestions that he had been duped: "I am just as certain I have not been duped as I am that certain scientists have been duped by the *Journal of the American Medical*

Association." When asked whether he had ever been wrong about anything in the past, Ivy flatly answered no.[53]

Durovic vehemently denied that Kositerin and Krebiozen were identical, and he shouted that it was "an insult" to ask him whether he had deceived Ivy. Allegedly, Durovic had packaged Krebiozen in mineral oil and glass ampules at his home in the Chicago suburb of Winnetka. He appeared to have ordered a substantial excess of mineral oil, and when asked what had happened to it, Durovic replied that he had dumped it all down the sewer behind his house. Durovic also had ordered what seemed to be an excessive number of ampules. He said that they were stored in his laboratory in a dingy neighborhood west of the Chicago Loop. The hearing was temporarily recessed so that everyone present—lawmakers, attorneys, witnesses, and journalists—could reconvene at the cramped laboratory. They discovered that thousands of ampules could not be accounted for, just like the missing mineral oil. It lent credence to Bohrer's charges that Krebiozen was being smuggled out of the country and sold around the world.[54]

Humberto Loretani arrived from Argentina to testify against the Durovic brothers. He said that the brothers had not invested a single penny in the production of Kositerin; that Stevan had never bought thousands of horses as he had claimed but instead had bought only fifteen bulls; that Stevan had charged vast sums for injections of Kositerin; and that the Durovics had promoted Kositerin as a cure-all for heart trouble, loss of virility, and cancer. Stevan vociferously challenged Loretani's claims, while his brother Marko reportedly called Loretani an insulting name in Spanish.[55]

Stoddard testified as well, returning to Illinois from his new home in Princeton, New Jersey. Boyle claimed that Stoddard could not take an oath swearing to tell the truth because Stoddard was an atheist. (Apart from serving as Ivy's lawyer, Boyle—the former Cook County state's attorney—also was reportedly helping put Krebiozen in ampules for shipping to patients.) Despite Boyle's objections, Stoddard was sworn in, and he told the legislative committee about the U of I's sorry experiences with Krebiozen while again explaining the choices that he had made as president. Stoddard said that the university had played "a long shot" on the off chance that Ivy finally would be able to prove Krebiozen's worth, only to be stymied by the Durovics.[56]

By the time that Stoddard testified, it was December. The *Courier* published a morose headline: "Krebiozen Hearing to Go On and On." However, after a session in which Bohrer called Stevan Durovic a "quack," Durovic called Bohrer a "bum," and Ivy called Bohrer a "liar," the legislative committee finally decided that it had heard enough, and it began negotiations on ending the proceedings. Those negotiations dragged on into the new year, as the AMA and other Krebiozen opponents complained that they had not been given an adequate chance to rebut all the charges made against them. The AMA also submitted affidavits from six cancer clinics across the country saying that seventy-three of seventy-six patients who had been treated with Krebiozen had subsequently died. Finally, in March 1954, after a raucous seven-hour, closed-door meeting, the legislative committee issued a report absolving everyone of conspiracy charges and also absolving Ivy and the Durovics of any wrongdoing. The report's only negative comment was aimed at Stoddard, who was said to have been guilty of "untactful handling of his public statements."[57]

The committee report also recommended further study of Krebiozen, which Ivy welcomed. He called on the AMA and the U of I to help conduct such a study, an idea that the AMA and the university both promptly rejected. Acting U of I president Lloyd Morey explained that the edict against further university involvement with Krebiozen still stood. That edict would remain in effect after David Henry became the new university president in 1955, and it never would be rescinded. Untactful or not, in issuing his decree against Krebiozen, George Stoddard had given the U of I a lasting gift.[58]

Although Stoddard had helped extricate the U of I from the drug, he was less successful in extricating himself. Far from subsiding after the Illinois legislative hearings, the Krebiozen controversy was about to expand across the country, and, once again, Stoddard would play a central role.

CHAPTER 4

A Fair Test

After losing his university presidency, George Stoddard professed to be at peace. "I've never felt so free in my life," he told reporters. He proudly pointed to the accomplishments during his seven years as head of the University of Illinois, including the vast increases in degrees granted and in appropriations obtained, the development of the betatron and the ILLIAC computer, the creation of institutes for the study of government and labor and communications, and the expansion of the renowned university library. To Coleman Griffith, who similarly had been ousted, Stoddard told of his happiness about moving to Princeton, New Jersey, where his family would be close to many old friends. "It is indeed with a sense of the carefree and the uncommitted that we move from heavy weights and other complexities with practically no responsibility and a delightful simplicity," Stoddard wrote to Griffith in August 1953.[1]

Behind his cheerful exterior, Stoddard was anxious. Unlike Griffith and Andrew Ivy, he had not held a tenured faculty position to which he could return after being removed from his administrative post. "I did not know where congenial work was to be found, and late summer was a poor time for a man of fifty-six to go job hunting in academic circles," he would recall. In addition, Stoddard was once again angry. He wrote sardonically to Griffith of "the midnight ride of Paul Revere Livingston," referring to the Board of Trustees president whom Stoddard blamed for his late-night forced resignation. He also blamed Illinois governor William Stratton, who, according to Stoddard, was plotting to seize control of the entire state "lock, stock, and barrel" by employing "the same kind of infiltration that enabled Hitler." (New U of I president David Henry would establish markedly better relationships with Stratton and with previously antagonistic trustees; to them, Henry offered the abiding advantage of not being Stoddard.)[2]

Stoddard said that he was offered a professorship in psychology at Princeton University, but he declined it. Despite being "inwardly furious" over his ouster, he was "still intellectually and emotionally tied to the University of Illinois," and he felt "deprived of any sense of closure: Illinois was unfinished business." He thus decided to set down for posterity how he had lost his U of I job over a phony cancer drug. Stoddard commandeered the dining room table in the small ranch house that his family was renting, and he began to write, pausing to return to Illinois on a couple of occasions to pore over a million words of sworn testimony from the state legislative hearings on Krebiozen. He received a four-hundred-dollar advance from Harcourt, Brace and Company for his manuscript, which was provisionally titled *The Great Krebiozen Hoax*.[3]

Stoddard soon ran into difficulties. For the rest of his life, on the subject of Krebiozen, he would feel obligated "to take extraordinary pains to get the facts straight and the supporting documents properly attested. Only in this way can I restore the actuality of a series of events unique in education, if not in medicine." Stoddard's completed manuscript would include an appendix nearly as long as the rest of the book. It compiled multiple documents on Krebiozen that included portions of Ivy's original 1951 report presented at the Drake Hotel, letters to and from Ivy and the Durovics, excerpts of the many university statements and resolutions on the drug, and the report issued by the legislative committee after its hearings. Together, the documents presented a valuable historical record, but they did not necessarily make for riveting reading. Because Stoddard's original publisher believed that the manuscript would not sell, Stoddard returned his advance, and he reached an agreement instead with Beacon Press in Boston. New concerns arose over potential liability, starting with the word *hoax* in the title. The manuscript was renamed *"Krebiozen": The Great Cancer Mystery*. Stoddard feared that it read too much "like a documentary" and that it was "not only without anger; it is practically without the juices of life." He fought to keep some of his more pungent commentary in the book.[4]

The published book was milder in tone than Stoddard's private correspondence; it even was milder than some of his public pronouncements on Krebiozen as president. Still, his skepticism toward the drug and his frustration with Ivy and the Durovics were obvious. Stoddard dismissed the conspiracy charges leveled by the pro-Krebiozen forces and by Ivy in particular: "What Dr. Ivy professed to view as a 'conspiracy' was nothing but the insistence of responsible persons upon the maintenance of ethical standards." Ivy himself represented a "personal tragedy" in how he had increasingly come to depend on the Durovics while shunning his fellow scientists. Stoddard criticized Illinois lawmaker Roland Libonati for portraying the U of I as being "opposed to the people of the state—a distortion astounding to those of us who know that state universities exist only to serve the people by offering the best educational and research facilities." The ex-U of I president also questioned why Roman Catholics seemed to back Krebiozen and Ivy so strongly, especially since Ivy was not Catholic himself; at the height of the Stoddard-Ivy standoff, Bishop Bernard Sheil had awarded Ivy the Pope Leo XIII Award. As Stoddard put it, "cancer, medical research, and university administration are *not* sectarian matters." He concluded by quoting the witches from Shakespeare's *Macbeth*: "eye of newt and toe of frog, wool of bat and tongue of dog." Stoddard wrote that "even at the end of the public legislative hearings, we knew more about the ingredients of the witches' brew than we did of the composition of 'Krebiozen'."[5]

Ivy and his lawyer John Sembower learned of Stoddard's book before it was completed, and they pushed to get *hoax* dropped from the title. However, they were hardly satisfied. "This book employs the Stoddard method of character assassination which is to employ the academic refinements of sarcasm, snobbish deprecation, and the dark innuendo," Sembower wrote to Ivy in March 1955 after reviewing the galleys. The lawyer thought that the book was defamatory, but he added that it might be difficult to prove libel; one Chicago attorney whom Sembower approached about helping to represent Ivy in a libel action refused the case, believing it to be weak. Sembower also told Ivy that seeking an injunction to prevent publication altogether risked raising "in the minds of some (often unjustly, to be sure) that the one bringing suit is afraid of what may be said or is trying to suppress matters." Yet Ivy believed that allowing himself to be defamed by what he called "lies" and then suing for damages was "only a flimsy and fanciful substitute for justice. After the horse is stolen and slaughtered, what good is it to collect damages to buy a lock for the barn door, especially when there is little or no horse or only a carcass to put in the barn?"[6]

Consequently, Ivy, the Durovics, and the Krebiozen Research Foundation sought a temporary restraining order in Boston blocking the publication of Stoddard's book. A judge granted the order in April. The action horrified free speech advocates, much as Sembower had warned. "Restraint prior to publication is the most vicious form of censorship, held to be unconstitutional a quarter of a century ago by the United States Supreme Court," the *Chicago Tribune* editorialized. *Publisher's Weekly* called the case "one of the most frightening for publishing in recent years." After vigorous legal challenges from Beacon Press, the injunction was lifted in July. Ivy then promptly sued Stoddard for libel, seeking $360,000 in damages even before the book was published in the fall. Beacon Press tried to take advantage of the publicity by promoting what the publisher described as "THE BOOK THEY COULDN'T BAN," but, according to Stoddard, Ivy's allies pressured bookstores not to stock it. As for Ivy's libel suit, because of various delays and failed attempts at an out-of-court settlement, it would be another six years before the case finally would go to trial.[7]

In the meantime, Krebiozen would seize the imaginations of a growing number of people across the country. It did so partly through the controversy generated by Stoddard's book, and even more so through a rival book that would shout Krebiozen's praises while damning Stoddard and everyone else who stood in the drug's way.

• • •

The rival book's author, Herbert Bailey, had had an unremarkable though diverse early career. An Atlanta native, he worked in the South as a journalist and a radio station promotion manager. He also spent several years in Chicago as a reporter; a critic for *Billboard* magazine; a publicist for the Walgreen Drug Company, the National Safety Council, and other organizations; and a writer of radio plays and stage plays. One of his plays was said to be "the story of what might happen in a totalitarian America ten years from now."[8] After World War II, Bailey carved out a niche as a science and medicine writer for popular magazines. He wrote about dental health for *Better Homes and Gardens*, ultrasound for *Science Digest*, and brain cancer diagnostic technologies for *Collier's*. On occasion, he seemed uncritical toward what certain sources were telling him, as when he wrote of how palm reading could help detect disease.[9]

In 1951, Bailey profiled seventy-six-year-old Émil Grubbé as being "one of our greatest medical heroes" for having developed X-ray therapy to treat cancer. Bailey would boast that he was responsible for ensuring that Grubbé "was finally accorded the recognition due him by the medical profession." In reality, according to a later biography of Grubbé, the scientist was prone to self-glorification and exaggeration of his achievements, and he furthered those ends through "a torrent of sympathetic, nondocumented newspaper and magazine stories," including Bailey's. Yet Bailey would say that Andrew Ivy saw his article about the scientific community's supposed neglect and mistreatment of Grubbé. The article encouraged Ivy to contact Bailey in July 1952 and share with the writer the report that Ivy had amassed on five hundred cancer patients treated with Krebiozen. "Judging from your articles and from my personal knowledge of you, you have always searched for and reported the truth," Bailey remembered Ivy telling him. "The falsity of the reports concerning Krebiozen and the baseness of the rumors concerning me and the discoverers of Krebiozen must be made known."[10]

Bailey, who already had been thinking about writing a book on Ivy, was converted. Krebiozen became his cause and his mission. "The people of the world and the world's doctors deserved to know the truth about a drug that showed more promise than anything medicine had yet discovered toward a solution of the most feared disease afflicting mankind," he would write. "They deserved to know the incredible behind-the-scenes actions which posterity may call the most sordid scandal of modern history." Bailey became a publicist for the Krebiozen Research Foundation, and, at the December 1952 U of I Board of Trustees meeting, he urged on Roland Libonati and other state lawmakers as they raucously praised Ivy and denounced Stoddard. Bailey even claimed credit for helping launch the state legislative hearings on Krebiozen, with the assistance of an unnamed friend (likely Effie Alley, who had worked with Bailey on the *Chicago Herald-American* and who, like Bailey, had become an advocate for Ivy and Krebiozen). Bailey handed out copies of pro-Krebiozen statements to reporters during the hearings. He also probably helped compile and distribute a pamphlet titled *False Witness* that used testimony from the hearings to try to discredit the negative reports on Krebiozen from the American Medical Association and the U of I's Cole Committee.[11]

By 1953, Krebiozen was drawing attention from nationally syndicated columnist Drew Pearson as well as from the US Congress. Pearson prided himself on defending individuals like Ivy who he thought were being mistreated by powerful people. He related in his column the "heartbreaking story" of "how New Hampshire's crusading Sen. Charles Tobey, on his own deathbed," sent Krebiozen "to his dying friend, Robert Taft. Senator Taft's doctors did not use it." Pearson wrote that fellow senators Arthur Vandenberg and Brien McMahon had benefited from Krebiozen, although both of them still had died from cancer. Pearson also reported that, prior to his death, Tobey had used Senate money to hire an investigator to scrutinize charges that the "doctors' lobby" was suppressing promising cancer treatments. The investigator, Benedict Fitzgerald, submitted his report to Congress in the summer of 1953. He accused the AMA of being "hasty, capricious, arbitrary, and outright dishonest," and he said that Krebiozen had fallen victim to "the weirdest conglomeration of corrupt motives, intrigue, selfishness, jealousy, obstruction, and conspiracy that I have ever seen." It was not only Krebiozen that was being squelched, according to Fitzgerald; so too were Harry Hoxsey's cancer treatment and William Frederick Koch's Glyoxylide. In light of the obvious limitations of radiation and surgery in curing cancer, surely those other treatments should receive further study:

especially Krebiozen, which, unlike Hoxsey Therapy and Glyoxylide, was not being sold for profit. Fitzgerald issued his report before Ivy announced that Krebiozen's promoters had begun requesting a nine-dollar-fifty-cent donation per ampule.[12]

Bailey would expand on Pearson's and Fitzgerald's writings as well as *False Witness* in writing his own book that was awkwardly titled *K, Krebiozen— Key to Cancer?* It was published by Hermitage House in early 1955 after Bailey pushed to release it before Stoddard's book appeared. (Hermitage House had previously published L. Ron Hubbard's book *Dianetics*, which gave rise to Scientology.) A revised and updated version of Bailey's book appeared three years later with a more provocative title—*A Matter of Life or Death: The Incredible Story of Krebiozen*—and with a more established

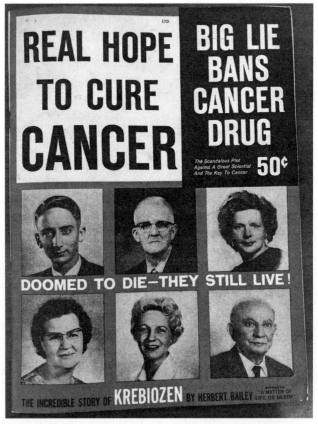

Cover of a pro-Krebiozen magazine written by Herbert Bailey. His book *A Matter of Life or Death* became the bible of the pro-Krebiozen movement. (Courtesy of the Chicago History Museum)

publisher, G. P. Putnam's Sons. A paperback edition followed in 1964. Bailey's book became the bible of the pro-Krebiozen movement and would help sustain that movement for years.[13]

If Ivy's friends compared him to Louis Pasteur, Bailey compared himself to Émile Zola, another great historical figure who, like Pasteur, had been portrayed by Paul Muni in a 1930s Hollywood movie. Bailey began his book by quoting Zola: "If you shut up truth and bury it under the ground, it will but grow, and gather to itself such explosive power that the day it bursts through it will blow up everything in its way." In an author's statement publicizing the book, Bailey noted that although Zola had been exiled for his incendiary 1898 essay "J'Accuse . . . !" that defended Alfred Dreyfus against the French military establishment, in the end, Dreyfus and Zola were both vindicated. Bailey saw his book as his own "J'Accuse . . . !" that defended Ivy and Krebiozen against the US medical establishment with similar faith in ultimate vindication.[14]

In the book, Bailey wrote that "the history of so-called 'cancer cures' teaches that one cannot be too overcautious in issuing claims and thereby engendering false hopes in both the medical profession and the general public." The biggest problems in the past had come not from obvious quacks, but instead from well-meaning and well-respected professionals who "were either misguided or unscientific or read their data wrong. Yet they believed in their product. And therein lies the danger of advancing any anti-cancer agent to the profession or to the public without strict objective proof of its efficacy."[15] Having made that acknowledgment, Bailey rejected any notion that Ivy had been misguided or had read his data wrong, nor did Bailey entertain any suggestion that the Durovics might have been less than forthright in their dealings. To him, Ivy and the Durovics stood unambiguously for science and truth; those individuals who challenged them stood unambiguously for avarice and falsehood.

Bailey charged the AMA with having pressured Lankenau Hospital in Philadelphia into stopping its use of Krebiozen after it initially reported good results with the drug. He also elaborated the case against the AMA's anti-Krebiozen reports. It did appear as though the AMA may have been sloppy or hasty in some of its findings. According to Ivy's testimony at the Illinois legislative hearings, Dr. Henry Szujewski—who in 1952 had published a report critical of Krebiozen in the *Journal of the American Medical Association*—had not personally seen some of the patients included in that report; he also had relied heavily on patients treated by Dr. William Phillips, who said that Szujewski had failed to report improvements that the patients had experienced with Krebiozen. The AMA had tried to get Phillips to list his name as a coauthor of Szujewski's *JAMA* article, but Phillips refused.

As for the original AMA report on Krebiozen published in October 1951, several of the patients whom the AMA said had died after taking the drug had been in the final stages of terminal cancer, and they had received only minimal doses. Bailey wrote that "it is hardly to be expected that many persons would rise from their death-beds and emerge cancer-free. *Yet that is the test* to which Krebiozen was subjected by research groups of the AMA, they knowing full well the impossibility of *any* agent accomplishing many miracles under these circumstances." A *New York Post* reporter who later examined the Krebiozen affair noted that the AMA had issued its report only a few months after Ivy's Drake Hotel meeting. "The AMA excuse for its unusual haste is that the razzmatazz which introduced the drug had created severe pressure to counsel besieged doctors," the *Post* reporter wrote. "That is plausible and may justify speed; nothing justifies shoddy data."[16]

Bailey also took aim at the U of I's Cole Committee report, again building on testimony from the Illinois Krebiozen hearings. He said that the Cole Committee had refused to examine closely a Krebiozen patient who, according to Bailey, had in fact "made a spectacular 'death-bed' recovery after she had been given up by all doctors." In addition, part of the committee's report containing personal patient information had not been released to the public, which Bailey said was significant because the unreleased portion contained positive findings about Krebiozen. For instance, the committee had examined a microscopic slide of a woman treated with the drug. Ivy's data stated that the woman still tested positive for cancer after taking Krebiozen, but the committee's review of the slide indicated that there was no cancer. The unreleased part of the Cole Committee report said that "this difference of opinion does not reflect disadvantageously on Krebiozen therapy, but might reflect advantageously."[17]

In another example, Ivy and his associates had presented to the committee thirteen patients who were said to display improvements after taking the drug. "Judged by this presentation alone, Krebiozen would appear to have beneficial effects," the unreleased part of the report said, adding that "no opinion of any kind can be expressed concerning these patients until after a period of several months." But Bailey charged that the Cole Committee still had rushed to issue a negative assessment of the drug in the public part of its report, much as the AMA had done. Bailey also criticized the committee for saying that the mystery surrounding Krebiozen's composition and manufacture should be dispelled; as Bailey put it, "thousands of drugs were (and are) used very effectively without the prescriber possessing the slightest knowledge of their history or their chemical make-up."[18]

The Cole Committee defended itself in language that was stronger than what it had used in its original report. According to the committee, scientists were obligated to know the nature of their experimental material at least to the degree that they could "repeat and verify" their experiments; in Krebiozen's case, "this simple scientific and humanitarian rule has been violated." The drug's promoters were "in the untenable moral position of withholding from the most prompt scientific testing channels, and thus possibly from many cancer patients, a compound which they claim has beneficial effect" on cancer. The failure to use a control group to compare people who had taken the drug with people who had not taken the drug also was inexcusable, particularly in testing a substance of "dubious value" such as Krebiozen. The Cole Committee declared that the original, public portion of its report accurately represented the committee's overall negative evaluation of the medicine.[19]

The AMA did not similarly defend itself, at least not publicly. In response to a doctor's query why the association was not being more vocal about Krebiozen, the AMA's Oliver Field replied that the association had regularly been the target of the likes of Norman Baker, Hoxsey, and Koch; the Krebiozen supporters' attacks were nothing new. Field said that AMA representatives including JJ Moore had been given no opportunity to defend themselves before the Illinois legislative committee, except indirectly during the AMA attorneys' cross-examination of Ivy and Stevan Durovic. Ivy's charges that the AMA had falsified its earlier anti-Krebiozen reports were untrue. Even so, the AMA was unwilling "to defend itself against each accusation as it crops up in books or pamphlets either sponsored by or inspired by the Krebiozen group. It is our position that no conspiracy ever existed, but for us to prove that would involve costly and long-drawn-out litigation."[20]

Bailey may well have wanted the AMA and other Krebiozen opponents to sue him for libel, much as Zola was said to have made his "J'Accuse . . . !" as inflammatory as possible to provoke French officials into suing him. A lawsuit against Bailey would have forced the anti-Krebiozen contingent into court where the conspiracy charges could be hurled anew, while also generating more publicity for the drug. As it was, Bailey applauded Ivy's libel action against Stoddard; he had urged Ivy to sue the AMA as well.[21]

Bailey also heaped invective on Krebiozen opponents in his book. The fact that the AMA had not testified on its own behalf during the legislative committee hearings essentially proved that the conspiracy existed; the committee's findings of no conspiracy were meaningless. The head of the U of I Tumor Clinic, Danely Slaughter, was implicitly linked to the conspiracy through his friendship with Ed Moore, one of the businesspeople accused of trying to steal Krebiozen. (Bailey targeted Slaughter because of his contributions to the AMA's negative report on the drug in 1951.)

Former U of I medical dean Stanley Olson was called "the loudest, most anguished breast-beater of them all" for having written letters criticizing Ivy. The Cole Committee's conclusions were said to "deserve a special place in the Archives of Cleverness, Smugness, and Piousness." Ivy's mentor, Anton Carlson, who could not fathom his former pupil's devotion to Krebiozen, was dismissed as a "once-thundering demander for the evidence" who in his declining years had failed to accept irrefutable proof of the drug's efficacy. The U of I was blasted for its "cowardly" refusal to overturn Stoddard's edict against Krebiozen after he left the university. As for Stoddard himself, Bailey viewed him as "a vain, egotistical man" who had been "more outspokenly rabid than the worst *medical* foes Krebiozen had ever encountered, or is still encountering." Stoddard was incensed over Bailey's book, which he privately called "incompetent" and error-ridden, but he resisted making his own book a rejoinder to Bailey's tome. For Stoddard, everything that the pro-Krebiozen forces did—including Ivy's libel suit against him—was calculated to discourage critical scrutiny of the drug and make money from it.[22]

In contrast, Bailey believed that he was on the side of the angels. He proclaimed that "unlike Zola, I do not now fight alone," and that "also unlike Zola, we have the scientific facts, facts which are provable *specifically*."[23] Krebiozen's proponents would come to include writers, doctors, celebrities, union members, advocates for nonmainstream medicine, and cancer patients and their family members, all of whom joined in common cause. They sought to blend science and passion in molding opinion and influencing policy on the drug. If the AMA could not be budged from its stance against Krebiozen, perhaps other representatives of organized medicine could be swayed differently.

• • •

The pro-Krebiozen writers included journalist Wade Jones, who published a pamphlet in early 1955 at about the same time that Bailey's book appeared. Like Bailey, Jones relied heavily on Ivy and the Durovics in making the case for a conspiracy against the drug. Jones did include a couple of quotes from other sources casting doubt on how well the drug actually worked and how venal the purported conspirators actually were. John Pick, one of the doctors who had been working with Ivy in testing Krebiozen, asserted that the drug could dissolve malignant tumors so quickly that it could boomerang on the patient by producing organ collapse or massive hemorrhaging. As Pick puzzlingly described one such case, "The patient was getting well, and so he died." Jones also quoted an affidavit from the AMA's Paul Wermer, who was present at the tense meeting in which the

Durovics charged AMA treasurer JJ Moore with maliciously interfering in their business affairs. According to Wermer, Moore told him after the meeting that if the Durovics were lying about their business ties, "they may be lying to Andy [Ivy] about what is in Krebiozen, or whether there is such a thing as Krebiozen, and I don't want to see Andy made the fall guy."[24]

Jones asserted that he was forced to pay to print his Krebiozen story in pamphlet form after "seven leading magazines, eight newspapers, and two feature syndicates" refused to publish it. He blamed AMA pressure for his inability to find a news outlet. Drew Pearson used his column to amplify Jones's charges of censorship while also pointing to another such case: *Clubwoman*, the magazine of the General Federation of Women's Clubs, had abruptly withdrawn its offer to publish an article by Ivy on Krebiozen, again supposedly because of the AMA. Pearson quoted *New York Times* science writer William Laurence as saying that "the AMA and the National Research Council have lied and been dishonest about krebiozen. The state of cancer research in this country today is a national crime."[25]

Ivy collaborated with Pick and William Phillips in making the scientific case for the drug in their book *Observations on Krebiozen in the Management of Cancer*, published in 1956. "Every physician and student of cancer in man knows that the medical literature has occasionally recorded the recession of malignant tumors after the administration of some form of medical therapy," they wrote. "Such a history should engender not a barren skepticism, but a zeal to discover the reason why and with what frequency these recessions occur." The authors said that when surgery and radiation did not work, "other palliative[s] and better therapy should be searched for." Krebiozen showed promise in buttressing the body's natural defenses against cancer and in offering an alternative to people who had not benefited from other treatments. Ivy and his associates reported that the drug had produced palliative effects in 68 percent of patients and reduced tumor size in 50 percent of them. Although many times the effects were only temporary, the authors speculated that it was because the drug was not administered in high enough doses. Some patients had survived for five years after starting Krebiozen. The authors did not believe that the positive results were attributable to the placebo effect or to other reasons independent of the drug. "*Of course, the only way that palliative effects can be established to the satisfaction of all critics is by the performance of a strictly controlled study entirely devoid of any possibility of bias on the part of the physician and patient,*" they underlined. "*This has never been done to our knowledge in the therapy of cancer in man, and we are anxious to do it in the case of Krebiozen.*"[26]

Observations on Krebiozen was published by Henry Regnery Company in Chicago, a conservative publisher that also had printed books by William

F. Buckley Jr. and by Robert Welch, who would soon found the John Birch Society. The Ivy-Pick-Phillips book was favorably reviewed in Buckley's new magazine *National Review* by Revilo Oliver, a U of I classics professor who would help Welch start the Birch Society. Oliver took a swipe at George Stoddard without naming him by asking whether "the little Hitlers who pullulate in the decay of our educational system have the right to dictate subjects of research to their professional serfs." Oliver added that the results reported in Ivy's book indicated "that further research with krebiozen is needed—and this, after all, is what Dr. Ivy claimed." Several years later, Oliver—who by that time had become a notorious conspiracy theorist, white supremacist, and anti-Semite—was invited to serve as master of ceremonies for a testimonial dinner honoring Ivy. It indicated that Krebiozen's supporters spanned the political spectrum and included individuals from both the fringe and the mainstream. Drew Pearson, who represented the mainstream news media, was Oliver's polar opposite in bitterly opposing such red-baiters as Joseph McCarthy.[27]

People with cancer who felt abandoned or abused by the medical establishment gravitated toward the drug. David Kasson, who began taking Krebiozen in 1956 after receiving surgery for what he was told was terminal cancer, was still alive a year later when he wrote a pamphlet titled "I Will Not Donate to the American Cancer Society." Kasson charged the ACS with "channeling donated funds to certain select organizations, apparently those controlled or beneficially used by the drug monopolies, and denying them to experienced, independent research scientists with the highest scholastic and scientific backgrounds." The ACS and the AMA were accused of conspiring to dominate US medicine with deadly consequences. "If a conspiracy exists, thousands of citizens have been deprived of their right to life and, if the evil is not corrected, millions more will be deprived of their lives in the future," Kasson wrote. In a separate essay, he declared that he never could stop taking Krebiozen, "any more than the diabetic can stop taking insulin. Though the Krebiozen Foundation sells at cost and seeks no profit, two weekly injections come to $19. Opposition of the AMA has prevented mass production methods which would bring the expense much lower."[28]

For a time, Kasson was part of a group called the Committee for Independent Cancer Research, which had been founded in Chicago in 1954 and which promoted both Bailey's book and the Ivy-Pick-Phillips book. The committee's chairperson was Gloria Swanson, the onetime silent movie icon who in 1950 had memorably starred as Norma Desmond in the film *Sunset Boulevard*. Swanson had lobbied for health foods and nonmainstream therapies for many years. In 1947, she had been diagnosed with a benign uterine tumor that she said she successfully treated by eliminating animal protein from her diet. While visiting her hometown of Chicago a few years later, she chanced to hear a radio commentator discussing the Krebiozen controversy. She read Bailey's book, agreed to chair the new pro-Krebiozen committee, and became arguably the most visible Krebiozen proponent in the country.[29]

Swanson appeared on the television show *This Is Your Life* in January 1957. After friends and former movie colleagues celebrated her on the show, she tried to work in a plug for Krebiozen; she later said that she was cut off before she could complete her appeal. She did receive a cash contribution from *This Is Your Life*'s producers for the Committee for Independent Cancer Research. A few months later, Swanson was the featured guest on a new ABC television program hosted by Mike Wallace, who already had cultivated an image as a take-no-prisoners interviewer. He quizzed Swanson about her support for what he called "an alleged cancer cure." Swanson

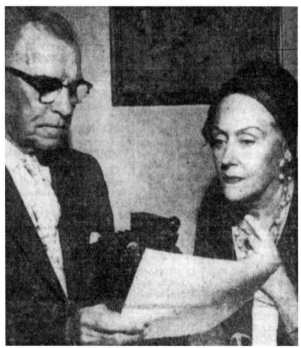

Gloria Swanson in the Lebanon, Pennsylvania, newspaper in September 1958. Swanson visited Lebanon to attend a lecture by Andrew Ivy. She is pictured with John Davis of the Committee for a Fair Test of Krebiozen.

calmly related the story of Andrew Ivy and Krebiozen, and she told of how David Kasson was apparently thriving thanks to the drug. She added that she hoped to raise enough money "to enable the top researchers in this country, and there are more than Dr. Ivy, to investigate any possible cure, or arresting, of cancer." When Wallace asked her where people could get more information, she replied that they could write to her directly at her home in Westport, Connecticut. Swanson received hundreds of letters in response to her television entreaties on behalf of her organization and Krebiozen.[30]

The following year, Kasson died. Herbert Bailey attributed his death not to cancer but to overwork, saying that Kasson had become "exhausted physically and emotionally by his ceaseless crusade" for Krebiozen. Before he died, Kasson had split from the Committee for Independent Cancer Research, which had grown unhappy over his repeated, agitated threats to sue the AMA and other agencies. The organization subsequently renamed itself the Independent Cancer Research Foundation. Swanson traveled on behalf of the organization to Lebanon, Pennsylvania, in September 1958, and she introduced a lecture that Ivy gave to an audience of nine hundred people. Bailey attended as well, bearing crutches and an ankle cast. He said that he had been mugged in New York, and he believed that he had been deliberately targeted because of his pro-Krebiozen activities. One of Bailey's friends later said that Bailey began carrying a gun after the mugging and "let it be known in AMA circles" that he was armed.[31]

Lebanon, Pennsylvania, had become a center of Krebiozen support largely because of Dr. Allen Rutherford, who had treated nearly one hundred patients with the drug by the time of Ivy's lecture in the city. Rutherford said that he had been denied access to a local hospital because of his use of Krebiozen. His wife wrote to Swanson that although Rutherford had suffered "slanderous comments, ridicule, and persecution from fellow practitioners," he remained devoted to the drug. He was convinced that conventional therapies did not work in the majority of cancer cases, and he believed that Ivy's drug gave the cancer patient comfort and relief, even if the patient ultimately died. As Rutherford's wife put it, Krebiozen allowed the doctor "to be able to give to another the privilege of passing on in his right mind and without pain."[32]

Three of Rutherford's Krebiozen patients were labor union members. They included John Schnelly, who belonged to the Lebanon Pressman Union, which printed the city's daily newspaper. Schnelly said that he had lived for five years on Krebiozen after doctors had told him that he had no chance of surviving his cancer. His union sponsored Ivy's lecture in Lebanon. Other labor groups took up Krebiozen's cause; they held little sympathy toward what the AFL-CIO Central Labor Council in Indianapolis called the "powerful financial interest of the A.M.A. and the tremendous influence that seems to follow naturally where money is used as the beckoning light." The Illinois Federation of Labor's executive vice president, whose wife had died of cancer, backed Ivy "in his struggle to get an honest scientific appraisal of krebiozen." The president of the Chicago Federation of Labor similarly pledged support. And Raymond Berndt of the United Auto Workers told members of his union that the apparent suppression of Krebiozen demanded collective action: "It is inconceivable to me that such a situation can continue to exist; so go out and build fires."[33]

In February 1959, the pro-Krebiozen coalition gathered in Chicago for a testimonial dinner for Ivy, one of many such fundraising dinners that would be held over the coming years. Among the twelve hundred attendees were Stevan Durovic; US senator Paul Douglas; Roland Libonati, now a member of the US House of Representatives; Gloria Swanson and Herbert Bailey; doctors John Pick, William Phillips, and Allen Rutherford; Park Livingston and John Boyle; Bishop Bernard Sheil; Chicago labor leaders Earl McMahon and Paul Iaccino; and several Krebiozen patients from across the country. Ivy told the audience that the existing supply of the drug would be exhausted by the summer, meaning that "those patients now dependent upon it will be left without it. Who then will be responsible for the consequences of taking away their Krebiozen? Not me, because I am going to work and appeal to others to help make a new batch." Saying that "no one will be able to rest in peace until the necessary funds are available," Ivy announced a fund-raising goal of $350,000.[34]

Like many other things about Krebiozen, the finances of the chief promoters of the drug were murky. One observer wrote of the Krebiozen Research Foundation in 1959 that "no extended report of the foundation's income, or the disbursement of its funds, has been made public." Stevan Durovic did release figures from the foundation's 1957 tax return indicating that expenses far outweighed income. He claimed that he had spent more than $82,000 of his own money on the drug since 1951, and he was running out of cash: "I'll be broke. This is what my enemies want." As for all the nine-dollar-fifty-cent donations that Krebiozen's promoters were requesting for the drug, Durovic said that the money was only enough to cover the cost of the drug's production. Ivy would say that the government regarded the Krebiozen Research Foundation as engaging in commercial product research because the name "Krebiozen" had been trademarked by the Durovics. As a result, donations to the foundation were not tax-deductible.[35]

To ensure that funds would be available to continue his research—and, perhaps, to distance himself somewhat from Durovic—Ivy set up a new organization separate from the Krebiozen Research Foundation. It was called the Ivy Cancer Research Foundation, and it performed research not on Krebiozen, but on a generic equivalent that Ivy called "lipopolysaccharide C." Ivy said that he had experimented with forty horses on a farm northwest of Chicago and had generated ten times the substance that Durovic claimed to have generated in Argentina from the same number of horses. According to Ivy, the substance that he had independently produced was chemically identical to Krebiozen. It was not clear whether this was the same substance that Ivy was now calling lipopolysaccharide C, or how much of it was going to desperate cancer patients at a time when the supply of Krebiozen was said to be almost depleted. At about this same time, Ivy published an article in a veterinary journal saying that he had successfully used a Krebiozen-like drug to treat cataracts in dogs.[36]

Notwithstanding, in comparison with Durovic, Ivy seemed to be taking the high road. Donations to his new foundation would be tax-deductible and would come through the help of local Ivy Cancer Leagues formed across the country. Ivy stated that he would earn no money from lipopolysaccharide C, that he would make public all his methods and findings, and that he would distribute the substance purely for scientific and charitable purposes. In contrast, Durovic's main goal seemed to be recouping the money that he and his brother claimed to have invested in Krebiozen. When the Independent Cancer Research Foundation held a fund raiser in New York in 1959 with Ivy and Gloria Swanson in attendance, the foundation's Dorothea Seeber told Swanson that a benefactor had donated one thousand dollars to go directly to Ivy for his research. "Please say nothing of this," said Seeber to Swanson, "as it must be slipped to Dr. Ivy without Dr. Durovic knowing it."[37]

Ivy stressed that he had not broken with Durovic. He continued to call for a fair test of Krebiozen—the trademarked drug—as opposed to his own substance, because it was "the fair thing to do" in the spirit of "American Free Enterprise." John Davis, the president of a Chicago construction company, headed both the Ivy Cancer Research Foundation and a group called the Committee for a Fair Test of Krebiozen until he died of a heart attack in 1960. Yet another pro-Krebiozen group, the Citizens Emergency Committee for Krebiozen, was based in New York. Its leaders included Rhoda Boyko, who was described by the press as a "Central Park South matron"; her family was known for its philanthropy toward Israel. Another leader was advertising executive Robert Marks, who had paid for a full-page *New York Times* ad promoting Herbert Bailey's book. The committee published a regular bulletin extolling the drug. "We do not want to see happen, ever again, what has happened in the case of Krebiozen," the bulletin declared in June 1960. "For if the truth about Krebiozen is longer denied the World, one must surely be fearful for the concepts called freedom, democracy and Christian-Judaic ethics." That same year, Herbert Bailey wrote a sixty-four-page pulp magazine on behalf of the drug. Its cover featured portraits of six Krebiozen patients and the headline "DOOMED TO DIE—THEY STILL LIVE!" Vilifying "the medical powers that be," Bailey promised that the day would soon come when Ivy would "smite them down with scientific truth, righteousness and wrath."[38]

Much of the news media seemed skeptical of such inflamed rhetoric. The *New York Post*, which published a six-part series on Krebiozen in 1960, wrote that "if Stevan Durovic has indeed discovered in Krebiozen the 'key to the control of cancer,' as his backers claim, it is a little like a high school physics teacher smashing the first atom all alone in his cellar." The *Post* also quoted one of Ivy's closest collaborators, Dr. William Phillips, about the alleged nefarious plot to crush Krebiozen: "That conspiracy stuff is for the birds." But the *Post* still advocated an objective test of the drug's worth through some agency of organized medicine. Other newspapers also backed a test, including the *Chicago Daily News* (which had grown increasingly dubious about Krebiozen), and even the *Chicago Tribune* (which had been dubious about the drug all along). Their logic was simple: the controversy had been dragging on for years, and it was long past time to resolve it. If the drug was shown to work, people should have easy access to it. If it did not work, it should no longer be made available. That was what Ivy, Durovic, and other Krebiozen proponents had been calling for all along—a definitive test that, if the results were positive, would finally enable the drug to gain scientific acceptance and allow it to be sold commercially.[39]

Arranging such a test would not be easy. There were ongoing disputes over which agency held jurisdiction over Krebiozen and which agency should test it. There also was the lingering question of just what Krebiozen was.

· · ·

From the start, Ivy had believed that Krebiozen was a hormone secreted by the reticuloendothelial system to fight disease. The US Department of Health, Education, and Welfare disagreed: it maintained that as a blood derivative, Krebiozen was a serum. The distinction was crucial, for whereas hormones were regulated by the Food and Drug Administration, serums were regulated by the Public Health Service. Congress had given the PHS authority over such vaccines as diphtheria antitoxin, which originally had been developed by infecting horses and then drawing their blood, much as Krebiozen was said to have been developed. At the time that Krebiozen emerged, the FDA and PHS differed in their criteria for granting a license that allowed a medicine to be sold. The FDA required only that the medicine be proved to be safe, whereas the PHS required that the medicine be proved to be both safe and effective. In addition, negative FDA rulings were open to appeal in court; negative PHS rulings were not.[40]

For obvious reasons, Ivy and Durovic wanted the FDA to hold jurisdiction over Krebiozen. Proving its safety seemed an easy hurdle—no one, not even the drug's biggest skeptics, had ever suggested that it was toxic. What was more, Ivy was genuinely convinced that Krebiozen was not an antitoxin like diphtheria vaccine but instead was a hormone; he had discovered many such hormones in his long career as a physiologist. The fact that the government refused to be similarly convinced suggested to Ivy and Durovic that the AMA may have pressured the government into giving the PHS authority over the drug and forcing Krebiozen to clear the much higher hurdle of demonstrating efficacy as well as safety. For the time being, the drug continued to be distributed to doctors for what was termed investigational use. Often the doctors requested the drug only because their patients had begged them for it. The doctors were supposed to return survey forms to the Krebiozen Research Foundation reporting their experiences with the medicine, but many times they failed to complete the forms. Krebiozen's promoters kept soliciting donations of nine dollars and fifty cents per ampule, since they held no license to sell the drug. Because they still wanted the license and Krebiozen still seemed to be under the PHS's oversight, the drug's promoters also kept pushing for a test to try to prove that it actually worked.[41]

But who would conduct the test? Both the AMA and the University of Illinois, where Ivy continued to be employed, had made it abundantly clear that they wanted nothing more to do with trying to evaluate Krebiozen. The drug's supporters turned instead to the American Cancer Society, which David Kasson already had attacked for its ostensible collusion with the AMA in quashing the drug. Still, the ACS wrote to Ivy in the fall of 1957 indicating that it was at least willing to talk about a possible test. The Krebiozen Research Foundation made a formal proposal early the following year. An evaluating committee of physicians and laypersons would be formed, with the foundation and the ACS each allowed to select members. The committee would evaluate one hundred people with cancer, half of whom would receive Krebiozen and half of whom would receive pure mineral oil. Only the laypersons would know which half had received the drug when it came time to compare the two groups of patients.[42]

Negotiations with the ACS over the proposed test soon foundered, particularly over Ivy's insistence that he be one of the physicians on the evaluating committee. The ACS believed that Ivy's inclusion would make a truly objective test impossible. Making matters worse was testimony before a California state legislative committee investigating quackery. University of California scientist Paul Kirk, who had analyzed a sample of Krebiozen, told the committee in May 1958 that he had found "nothing more than pure Nujol—a laxative. In other words, it is a good grade of mineral oil and absolutely nothing else." Stanford University scientist Arthur Furst had analyzed his own Krebiozen sample, and he concurred with Kirk's assessment. Ivy, who had defended Krebiozen before the same legislative committee, bitterly attacked Kirk's and Furst's findings as being "demonstrably untrue" and as containing "astounding discrepancies," but his protestations did nothing to make the ACS more amenable toward participating in a test.[43]

In August 1958, Senator Paul Douglas presented his own test proposal. Again, half of a group of people with "more or less terminal cancer" would receive Krebiozen, and the other half would receive a placebo. Using terminal cases lessened the ethical concerns about withholding a hypothetical cancer remedy from half the group; presumably, everyone in the group already had received conventional therapies that had not succeeded in curbing their disease. Ivy would participate "in an advisory diagnostic and therapeutic capacity," although he would not know which patients had received Krebiozen. Rather than relying on the ACS to oversee the test, Douglas approached the National Cancer Institute and its head, John Heller. Douglas brushed aside Heller's suggestion that the drug should first be tested on animals: "May I say very frankly that what I am interested in and what I think vitally concerns the public is the problem of cancer in men, not in mice."[44]

The NCI was coming under significant pressure not only from Douglas but also from Krebiozen supporters nationwide who did not care which agency conducted a test as long as the test actually happened and it confirmed what they believed they already knew—Krebiozen was the key to treating cancer. The Committee for a Fair Test of Krebiozen and its chairperson, Zelma Lee Ross, reported in late 1958 that the committee had gathered more than a half-million signatures on petitions calling for a test. Joining the call were the Independent Cancer Research Foundation and the Prairie State Health Federation, the latter group being an Illinois affiliate of the National Health Federation; those organizations saw Krebiozen as vital to their broader agenda of gaining acceptance for nonmainstream health remedies. In response to the intense lobbying, the NCI's Heller cautiously ventured that evaluation of Krebiozen "should be explored further," while Douglas expressed hope that the impasse over a test finally would be broken.[45]

Douglas's optimism was unfounded. In March 1959, the NCI announced that it had rejected Ivy's conditions for a test. Ivy was said to go well beyond what Douglas had proposed by wanting to administer the drug himself and interpret the results himself, which struck the NCI as being outlandishly biased and unscientific. The American Cancer Society concurred and prepared what it called "A Background Paper on Krebiozen" that was published in the *Journal of the American Medical Association*. The ACS said that it held "the responsibility of seeing to it that the public is not misled by enthusiastic claims of individuals who would exploit unproven methods or drugs for the treatment of cancer," and it added that "no acceptable evidence that treatment with Krebiozen causes any objective benefit in human cancer has yet been offered by independent researchers."[46]

The Krebiozen Research Foundation responded by attacking both the NCI and the ACS in language that echoed previous broadsides against the AMA, the U of I, and the scientists who said that Krebiozen was nothing but mineral oil. "Dr. Heller's actions show that he, like the American Cancer Society, does not want a test that will establish the truth about Krebiozen, but only a chance to liquidate it," the foundation said of the NCI head. As for the ACS paper on Krebiozen, it was rife with "half-truths and falsities in order to discredit krebiozen and its supporters in the eyes of the public." ACS vice president Harold Diehl wrote to Paul Douglas that his organization would not bother trying to rebut the charges of the drug's proponents. "If they are sincere in their concern for the cancer patient, they should no longer insist that krebiozen be exempted from the procedures that are applied to all other substances," Diehl said. He added that he had had a long career in medicine, and "never in all these years did I encounter tactics such as have been used to promote krebiozen."[47]

Thus, by 1960, when the *New York Post* joined other newspapers in calling for a test of the drug, the prospects did not seem promising. However, in the fall of that year, Ivy and Durovic met with the new head of the NCI, Kenneth Endicott. Ivy and Durovic agreed to give the NCI data on forty-seven hundred Krebiozen patients to lay the groundwork for a test. "It's like working for 10 years and finally seeing a little light on the other side of the horizon," Ivy said. Anxieties about the diminishing supply of the drug were mollified after Durovic announced that he had manufactured a new batch using two hundred horses on a farm seventy miles from Chicago. Pictures of the horses and of Durovic in a white lab coat duly appeared in Herbert Bailey's pulp magazine promoting the drug. The pictures appeared under the headline "AMA-ACS Charge of 'secrecy' disproved by these photos!" The *Post* even published what it said was the exact chemical formula and production process of Krebiozen, having confirmed the information with

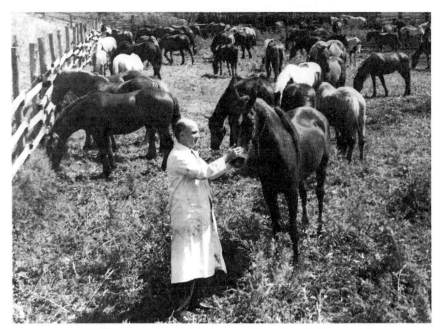

Stevan Durovic in 1960 alongside horses that he said he used to produce Krebiozen. The medicine's proponents insisted that this photo proved that there was nothing secret about the drug.

Ivy and Durovic. Three scientific experts told the newspaper that the formula would be reproducible in a laboratory, although one of them added that "I don't know how you'd know what you had when you got through."[48]

The biggest impetus yet for a test came in the spring of 1961, when Ivy's libel suit against George Stoddard finally came to trial in federal court in Chicago before Judge Julius Miner. Stoddard would remember that he and Ivy "sat tandem fashion beside a long table, ignoring each other." Believing that the jury could not determine whether Stoddard's book was defamatory without knowing its contents, the judge ordered that it be read aloud, a process that took four days. "In the quiet courtroom I tried to put myself in the place of a juryman and found myself silently convinced of the worthlessness of 'Krebiozen' and the reasonableness of my book," Stoddard recalled. Ivy told reporters outside the courtroom that he was prepared to call two hundred Krebiozen patients as witnesses. Although attorneys for both sides said that the effectiveness of Krebiozen was not the trial's primary concern, Judge Miner disagreed: "It is the vital issue." If Krebiozen was worthless as Stoddard had claimed in his book, then what he had written was true, and hence not libelous. The only way to prove whether Krebiozen was worthless, though, was through a test.[49]

Therefore, the judge recessed the trial and sent a letter to Abraham Ribicoff, the secretary of the Department of Health, Education, and Welfare. "In my humble judgment, Krebiozen has too long been a controversial subject and the American public deserves that it be examined under neutral supervision and by the most competent experts in whom the people have implicit confidence," Miner wrote to Ribicoff. "Needless to add that your Department and the National Cancer Institute under your supervision has the confidence of all the litigants and of this court." A few days later, Miner announced that the government had agreed to test Krebiozen. "The very fact that our national government has assumed this responsibility emphasizes the urgency for a public solution of this controversy," the judge said, adding, "There must be no quibbling, withholding, hindering, evading, or procrastinating in this test."[50]

In fact, the whole gamut of quibbling to procrastinating was still in store for Krebiozen. In time, the drug finally would be evaluated by the government, but not in the manner that Ivy wanted. The results would indicate that Stoddard had been right all along.

CHAPTER 5

Nothing but Creatine

By the time that his libel suit against George Stoddard came to trial in the spring of 1961, Andrew Ivy had turned sixty-eight years old, the mandatory retirement age at the University of Illinois. The faculty senate of the U of I's professional colleges in Chicago voted to discontinue the Department of Clinical Science, which had been specially created for Ivy when he was first hired. A College of Medicine committee had found that the department now had only three university staff members—Ivy, a research associate, and a clerk—and it had virtually ceased any undergraduate or graduate teaching. Ivy's impending retirement seemed the ideal time to fold his department and reallocate its space and resources to more pressing needs in the college.[1]

Ivy and his political allies had other ideas. Two Chicago lawmakers introduced bills in the Illinois legislature that would preserve Ivy's department with him still as its head and at the same time raise the university's retirement age to seventy. Ivy also would be given the option of staying on until age seventy-five. Lawmakers presented a separate resolution calling for Ivy to be given whatever he needed to continue his investigation of Krebiozen. In an outraged editorial, the *Chicago Daily News* questioned whether the university was "going to be directed by its administrators and its faculty, or by a group of legislators with political axes to grind and who couldn't distinguish between carcinoma and chow mein." Eventually, the pro-Ivy and pro-Krebiozen measures in the legislature were tabled. U of I president David Henry reminded the Board of Trustees that the university's Krebiozen ban imposed in 1952 by Stoddard still stood. Ivy's mandatory retirement and the discontinuance of his department would proceed as scheduled, but he would be granted emeritus status and provided lab facilities for another year to complete non-Krebiozen research projects.[2]

In the summer of 1962, as Ivy's additional year was drawing to a close, Roland Libonati made a final pitch to keep him at the U of I. Libonati had been Ivy's most vocal supporter in the Illinois legislature during the 1953 Krebiozen hearings; he subsequently was elected to the US Congress. Libonati wrote to President Henry that Ivy had devoted "the best years of his life and his research to the University of Illinois, and now to deny him this few square feet of space where he can finish his work for the benefit of Mankind, and which will reflect credit upon our great University, is a rather shabby way of treating a world-renowned scientist." Joseph Begando, the U of I vice president in charge of the Chicago professional colleges, sent his own letter to the university administration protesting any attempt to delay Ivy's departure. "We are doing everything possible to assist Dr. Ivy in the transition involved," Begando wrote, which was to say discreetly that they were keen on finally getting rid of him.[3]

Ivy ended up creating an entirely new position for himself. In July 1962, he wrote to Edward Sparling, the president of Roosevelt University, a private institution founded in 1945 in Chicago. Ivy told Sparling that he wanted to join Roosevelt's faculty. He would require no salary and would pay for any necessary facility renovations to accommodate his needs. With the support of the university's chemistry department, Ivy became a research professor of biochemistry at Roosevelt the following fall. It cost more than $23,000 to refurbish space for Ivy's laboratory, with the money coming from donations by the Ivy Cancer Research Foundation, the Krebiozen Research Foundation, and Ivy's friends.[4]

Ivy's lab was located in the tower of the historic Auditorium Building on Chicago's Michigan Avenue opposite Grant Park. The building, which had opened in 1889, had been designed by Louis Sullivan and Dankmar Adler, with Frank Lloyd Wright contributing as an apprentice. Roosevelt University had moved into the building in 1946. After Ivy began working in the tower, his friends nicknamed it the "Ivy Tower," and Ivy professed delight at being there. "My new facilities are very good; in fact, the best I have ever enjoyed except at Northwestern where I had the best in the world in 1946," he wrote to Joseph Begando in early 1963. The implication was that he had been forced to make do with barely adequate facilities during all of his years at the U of I.[5]

According to legend, the Auditorium Building was haunted. People claimed that they heard mysterious voices at night in the tower, where Sullivan, Adler, and Wright had once occupied an office; the voices were said to be those of the architects quarreling into eternity. A wraithlike aura also hung over Ivy's laboratory. One Roosevelt student recalled seeing a collection of cadaverous visitors regularly entering and departing the lab, presumably people with late-stage cancer who were grasping at one last chance for life. The student described it as "a parade of doomed hopefuls."[6] Perhaps in a small way Ivy subconsciously identified with them. Although he maintained a brave face, by the time that he took occupancy in the tower, his hopes for winning scientific acceptance of Krebiozen appeared similarly doomed.

• • •

It had been clear for some time that the government held significant reservations about testing Krebiozen the way that Ivy wanted. Even as Judge Miner had announced in April 1961 that the Department of Health, Education, and Welfare had agreed to a test, HEW's Abraham Ribicoff was telling Miner that Ivy and Stevan Durovic would first have to meet multiple conditions. The conditions were (1) the disclosure of complete information about Krebiozen's production and composition, (2) sufficient animal data to prove the drug's safety and indicate its potential value for human use, and (3) full data from physicians on their experiences with the drug over the previous ten years. "Any decision to undertake a study with human cancer patients must await, and depend on, the results of the evaluation of the existing clinical data," Ribicoff wrote to Miner. "We cannot agree to conduct or to encourage its investigational use in human patients, either in our own [agencies] or in other institutions, until we have first been furnished the scientific information which warrants such a step." The National Cancer Institute, which seemed the most likely agency to perform a test, was part of HEW, as were the Food and Drug Administration (FDA) and the Public Health Service (PHS).[7]

Ribicoff's letter highlighted intractable differences between Krebiozen's proponents and the government. Ivy was leery of having another group similar to the U of I's Cole Committee evaluate Krebiozen. As he put it, "we do not want the opinion of a committee; we want a fair test." For him, "fair" meant that he would be closely involved with the test, an idea that the government continued to reject as being biased. There also was a conflict over what was required to guarantee that the test would happen. Ivy and Durovic believed that once they delivered all the information that Ribicoff had requested, the test would proceed. As Ribicoff's letter noted, though, the government would use the information merely as a basis for deciding whether a test was even justified. Finally, a conflict remained over which agency held authority over Krebiozen. Again, the FDA at that time required only that a medicine be shown to be safe, whereas the PHS required that it be shown to be both safe and effective. Consequently, in 1954, Ivy and Durovic had submitted an official New Drug Application to the FDA, only to be told that the government considered Krebiozen to be a serum under the jurisdiction of the PHS. In the years that followed, Krebiozen remained in a gray area where it could be distributed for experimental use but without a license permitting its sale.[8]

In March 1961, Durovic tried once more for a license by sending another New Drug Application to the FDA. Three months later, the FDA deemed Durovic's application "incomplete and inadequate." The application had not fully reported animal data and human clinical data on the administration of the drug. It had not definitively shown that Krebiozen was safe to use; although no one had charged that the drug was toxic, the burden of proof remained on Durovic to demonstrate conclusively that it did no harm. The information provided was insufficient to establish the medicine's "identity, strength, quality, and purity." The FDA called it "most extraordinary" that the only information provided about the drug's composition had been derived from "incompletely described tests made on Krebiozen extracted from a dilution containing 0.01 mg. per ml. of mineral oil." Durovic had claimed that the drug was so remarkably potent that it could only be administered in a solution of one part Krebiozen to one hundred thousand parts oil. The FDA also said that available data did not support Durovic's assertion that the drug was a hormone falling under FDA jurisdiction. Durovic should therefore abandon his hopes for FDA approval and instead concentrate on winning the favor of the PHS.[9]

Apparently undaunted, Ivy, Durovic, and their colleague John Pick submitted a report to the National Cancer Institute in late September that summarized the results of Krebiozen as administered by some thirty-three hundred doctors across the country to some four thousand people with cancer. In addition, Ivy submitted a scientific manuscript to the *Journal of the National Cancer Institute* outlining those doctors' experiences with the drug. The NCI also announced that Durovic had provided the chemical formula for the drug along with ten milligrams of Krebiozen powder undissolved in mineral oil. Krebiozen's sponsors believed that they had met all of the government's stipulations for proceeding with a test.[10]

The government disagreed. The NCI journal rejected Ivy's manuscript, saying that it did not provide enough information to allow other scientists to replicate the research. The thirty-three hundred doctors did not appear to have used uniform procedures in administering the drug. The manuscript had not used statistical tests correctly, nor was it formatted properly. Then, in March 1962, NCI director Kenneth Endicott wrote to Ivy and Durovic that the cancer institute had completed its review of the data that Krebiozen's sponsors had submitted the previous September. "We are disappointed with what we found," Endicott said. It was hardly clear that the people who had taken Krebiozen had benefited from the drug, particularly since many of them had also received other treatments for their cancer; there was nothing to show whether their reported improvements were attributable to Krebiozen or to the other therapies. Once again, information was insufficient about the drug's use in animals and about the drug's production and composition. Although Durovic had given the NCI a bit of Krebiozen powder and the purported formula, they still were not enough to determine precisely what the drug was. "From the evidence available to us, we do not find a basis for any clear meaning of the term 'Krebiozen,'" Endicott wrote. He concluded by reiterating that the drug's sponsors as yet had failed to fulfill the conditions necessary for the NCI "to meet our scientific and moral responsibility. We will not sponsor a clinical trial until such conditions are met."[11]

Some NCI officials privately wondered whether the cancer institute was treating Krebiozen too harshly and asking more of the drug's sponsors than it did of sponsors of other treatments. Very likely, the NCI and other government agencies resented the political pressure put on them to test Krebiozen and the attacks they faced whenever they questioned the justifiability of a test. Krebiozen's most persistent political proponent—Paul Douglas—took to the US Senate floor in July 1962 to blast the NCI for its refusal to test the drug, and he suggested cutting its funding. Douglas accused the agency of having "fallen under the control largely of the pundits of the American Medical Association" and of being "ruled by the prejudices of organized medicine." Douglas also entered into the record a lengthy and combative letter that Ivy, Durovic, and Pick had sent to Endicott. "If we are denied knowledge of the individuals who have refuted our work; are denied publication of our findings in your scientific journal; and are denied an opportunity to demonstrate and discuss our findings with your scientists, we are frustrated in the face of the exercise of such arbitrary power," the letter said.[12]

However, the letter also implicitly acknowledged one of the biggest concerns that multiple agencies and committees had raised about Krebiozen over the years: the drug's sponsors were relying almost entirely on haphazard, secondhand information collected from doctors who had acquired the drug on behalf of patients who had asked or pleaded for it. Clinical data thus gathered on Krebiozen never would satisfy scientific protocol. The NCI wanted much more complete medical records on the people who had taken the drug, which was information that Ivy, Durovic, and Pick did not have. They suggested to Endicott "that the NCI obtain the services of other Federal agencies with the legal authority and power to secure this information from hospitals and physicians who have refused it to us."[13]

Another major concern that had been raised from the start about Krebiozen was that no one other than Durovic seemed to know what Krebiozen was or how it was made. A meeting that Senator Douglas brokered between Ivy and Endicott in September 1962 did little to clear up the confusion. Ivy repeated his claim that he had independently produced a substance that was chemically identical to Krebiozen, but he would not give any of it to the NCI. Durovic's Krebiozen continued to be the product that Ivy and Durovic wanted the NCI to test, not Ivy's lipopolysaccharide C, which was reserved purely for Ivy's own research. That arrangement, which supposedly honored Durovic's financial investment in Krebiozen, forced NCI officials to rely on Durovic to provide adequate samples of the drug and information about its production. Such cooperation from Durovic was not forthcoming. He had been deliberately excluded from the meeting with Endicott, and he responded by attacking the NCI anew. "Why is the NCI, as a representative of organized medicine, trying so desperately to avoid our challenge to test Krebiozen[?]," Durovic asked. "They are trying to avoid being placed in a situation where they would have to admit the worth of Krebiozen publicly. Such an admission would write *finis* to theirs [*sic*] and their allies' scientific authority."[14]

The intransigence of Krebiozen's sponsors encouraged the government to do exactly what the sponsors had suggested—find out directly from doctors and hospitals how Krebiozen was being used and what effects it was having on patients. Added impetus would come from Congress, which, at the instigation of Senator Estes Kefauver, had been holding long-running hearings on problems with drug regulation. During the hearings, Cornell University scientist Walter Modell leveled charges at the pharmaceutical industry that were virtually identical to the ones aimed at Krebiozen over the previous decade: the industry was guilty of "a short-sighted view of all the effects" of drugs, as well as "faulty experiments; premature publication; too-vigorous promotion; exaggerated claims and careless use—in brief, a break in the scientific approach."[15]

Kefauver's proposed legislation to strengthen federal drug laws had stalled in Congress. Then, in the summer of 1962, the *Washington Post* reported that FDA reviewer Frances Oldham Kelsey had almost single-handedly prevented the morning-sickness drug thalidomide from being sold in the United States. Kelsey had resisted significant pressure to approve the manufacturer's New Drug Application, because she believed that claims about the drug's safety had not been proved. In fact, thalidomide produced thousands of instances of birth defects in Europe and elsewhere in the world (including a number of cases in the United States after the drug's distributor recklessly dispensed it for trial and promotional purposes). The publicity generated by Kelsey and Thalidomide helped enact the Kefauver-Harris Amendment to the Federal Food, Drug, and Cosmetic Act in October 1962. Apart from now requiring manufacturers to demonstrate not just the safety but also the efficacy of a medication prior to FDA approval, the new legislation also closed a major loophole in the previous law, which had allowed a drug to be distributed for experimental use with few restrictions. The new law "stated that experiments on humans could not be done at will and without records," observed medical writer Philip J. Hilts. Experiments with new drugs "had to be 'adequate,' meaning large and numerous enough studies. They had to be 'well controlled,' meaning that testimonials and unverifiable results would no longer suffice. 'Controlled' meant studies that included comparisons of patients who took the treatment with those who did not."[16]

Krebiozen's promoters had been seeking federal approval of their drug on the basis of spotty patient records, uncontrolled studies, and testimonials of miraculous results with sparse supporting evidence. The fallout from Thalidomide and the enactment of the Kefauver-Harris Amendment gave the FDA new power and prestige to exert the scientific authority that Durovic seemed to mock and Ivy seemed to have forsaken. On January 15, 1963, the government announced that the FDA would lead a comprehensive government investigation of Krebiozen, including reports that the medicine was being illegally sold. The drug continued to be distributed for what were called "donations" of nine dollars and fifty cents per ampule.[17]

Three days after that announcement, Judge Julius Miner entered a Chicago hospital. It had been nearly two years since he had asked the government to test Krebiozen promptly and finally help resolve Ivy's libel suit against George Stoddard. That test still had not happened, and the libel suit still was not resolved. On March 13 Miner died, shocking colleagues who had not known how ill he was. The cause of death was cancer.[18]

• • •

The impending FDA investigation alarmed Krebiozen advocates and patients. Ivy and Durovic wrote to HEW official Boisfeuillet Jones that "several of these patients, the continuance of whose life has been found to be dependent on the hormone and/or drug, have frantically contacted us personally or through their attorney, seeking assurance that their lives would not be threatened by the withdrawal of Krebiozen." Ivy and Durovic did not seem inclined to assuage those people's mounting anxiety, which proved to be a potent tool in putting new pressure on the government to reverse course and ensure continued access to the drug.[19]

Prominent journalists came to Krebiozen's aid in 1963. In his syndicated column distributed across the country, Drew Pearson expressed sympathy for the people who believed that they could not survive without the medicine. Chicago newspaper columnist Jack Mabley devoted multiple articles to praising Ivy and calling on the government to accede to the kind of test that Ivy wanted. "If Krebiozen is not a fraud, then as many as a million lives may have been lost needlessly while this bickering has been going on. And a million more can be lost while it continues," Mabley told his readers. In Boston, columnist George Frazier waged a virtual crusade against the American Medical Association for its opposition to the drug. "The attitude of the AMA toward Krebiozen is one of the tragedies of our time—and perhaps of all other times as well," he wrote, while also accusing the AMA of playing "politics with human lives" and resorting to "the dirtiest of pool in an effort to brainwash its members."[20]

Journalists who otherwise took no strong stand on Krebiozen were quick to note that the drug's supporters could not all be dismissed as crackpots.[21] Some of the most devoted supporters were women of considerable accomplishment and civic commitment. Catherine Manning, the executive director of the Ivy Cancer Research Foundation, had been a founding member of the Women's Architectural League in Chicago and a board member of the American Association of Social Workers. Dorothea Seeber, a leader of the Independent Cancer Research Foundation, also would write a popular children's book. Gloria Swanson, of course, was a cinema icon in addition to being a vigorous proponent of nonmainstream medicine. By 1963, Swanson had begun to reduce her efforts on behalf of Krebiozen ("what more I can do God only knows," she had told one of the drug's supporters), but not before she had written to President John F. Kennedy urging him to intervene: "Since no visible prolongation of life without excruciating pain treatment has been found in what the AMA terms orthodox methods, I cannot see why Krebiozen cannot get a fair test, or far better, have a license for its use."[22]

Much of the support for Krebiozen stemmed from mainstream medicine's shortcomings. In asking for patience with cancer research, NCI director Kenneth Endicott acknowledged that "we have certainly not found a cure," and he added that although doctors had begun using a dozen new chemicals to treat cancer, they were not much better than previous therapies. One doctor would note that there was a "very rigid determinism" in cancer research that was prejudiced against new ideas about causes or treatments.[23] Women with cancer often felt victimized by the medical establishment, with good reason. Cecile Hoffman—who would found a group in 1963 called the International Association of Cancer Victims and Friends—wrote of being subjected to a radical mastectomy, which was standard procedure at the time. After the surgery, her cancer soon metastasized. "Medical doctors are only allowed to treat breast cancer within a set protocol, all radical, all mutilating, all expensive and very limited in restoring the victims to health," Hoffman said. Her ordeal would turn her toward nonmainstream cancer remedies.[24]

Rachel Carson's experience was similar to Hoffman's. A renowned marine biologist and ecologist, Carson already had begun writing *Silent Spring* when she underwent a radical mastectomy in 1960. Her surgeon told her only that she had "a condition bordering on malignancy." In fact, he had lied to her about her pathology reports—Carson had cancer that had metastasized. Such untruths were common among doctors at that time; they rationalized that they did not want to demoralize their patients.[25]

Carson, convinced that she had been subjected to "rather slap-dash" treatment and wanting "a more skilled judgment brought to bear on the problem," turned to Dr. George Crile Jr. Crile already had rejected radical mastectomies as being ineffective and needlessly disfiguring. He also had published a book in 1955 called *Cancer and Common Sense*. "If physicians, in an age that is thought of as being an age of science, devote themselves solely to the scientific side of medical practice, if they fail to inspire their patients with hope and faith, it is not surprising that quackery flourishes," he had written. Of course, Crile did not shun science. He was frank with Carson about the extent of her disease and recommended that she begin radiation therapy, which she undertook while completing *Silent Spring*. The groundbreaking book, which exposed certain pesticides' calamitous impact on the environment, was published in September 1962. It drew acclaim from readers and book critics as well as attacks from the chemical industry.[26]

By early 1963, it was obvious that Carson's cancer was continuing to spread. She decided to try Krebiozen, having researched it thoroughly. "It is an anti-cancer substance produced by living tissues," she wrote to her close friend Dorothy Freeman. "So, instead of attacking the local manifestations of the disease, as by radiation, it really helps the whole body resist." (Chemotherapy was still a relatively novel cancer treatment in the early 1960s.) Carson knew all about the controversy surrounding Krebiozen, but she blamed it on "chiefly the bickerings, struggle for power, bigotry, etc., within the medical profession rather than any valid objection to the drug." When she informed Crile of her plan to use the medicine, she similarly acknowledged "the AMA's longstanding war" against the drug, adding, "But then I have seldom if ever found myself in agreement with the AMA! Their attacks on Krebiozen resemble so closely some of the methods used against those critical of pesticides that the parallel is quite suggestive." Carson feared that Crile might object to her taking the drug, but true to what he had written in his book, he encouraged her to try whatever would help her maintain hope and faith. "I think the main thing in the treatment of this disease is to keep busy doing something," Crile wrote to Carson, "and certainly Krebiozen would be as good as anything else except hormones."[27]

Carson kept her health problems out of the public eye, but other women openly proclaimed their use of Krebiozen. Freda DeKnight had become food columnist for *Ebony* magazine in Chicago in 1946 and had written a book about African American cuisine called *A Date with a Dish* that would be republished in multiple editions. DeKnight also helped inaugurate the annual Ebony Fashion Fair, and she was one of the discoverers of Diahann Carroll, who started modeling for *Ebony* as a teenager. After being diagnosed with cancer in 1960, DeKnight underwent surgery and was frequently confined to a wheelchair; even so, she maintained a grueling work schedule. While on a trip to Asia in early 1962 to buy clothes for the fashion fair, she began taking Krebiozen, convinced that it was prolonging her life.[28]

Eighteen-year-old Diane Lindstrom also took the drug. In January 1963, the high school senior from Rockford, Illinois, received a shattering diagnosis: the leg pain that she had been experiencing was bone cancer. Her doctor recommended amputating her leg. Two days before the scheduled operation, the daughter of a hospital worker told Lindstrom's family about Krebiozen. Lindstrom decided to forego the amputation and try the medicine, with her parents acceding to her wishes. Andrew Ivy quoted her as saying that she "would rather die than go through life without a leg." Lindstrom herself noted that her "outlook was not too bright" even with an amputation; her doctor had said that it would give her only a one-in-five chance of surviving five years. After she started taking Krebiozen, her pain vanished and her tumor appeared to shrink, according to Ivy. The Rockford doctor who had recommended amputation challenged Ivy's claims and charged that using Krebiozen on the young woman was unethical; in return, Ivy accused the doctor of "professional jealousy." Lindstrom's embrace of Krebiozen received national news attention, and she received scores of letters of support from other cancer patients, college students, and even a detachment of Marines in Hawaii.[29]

Krebiozen's most dedicated advocate as of 1963 may have been Laine Friedman of Flushing, New York. She had long supported social and political causes, including the civil rights movement and the Women's International League of Peace and Freedom. In the spring of 1961, her husband George had been diagnosed with inoperable stomach cancer. "I resolved to fight this thing," she would recall. At her urging, a doctor reluctantly began administering Krebiozen, and, according to Friedman, her husband responded quickly and dramatically: "His appetite increased. He was able

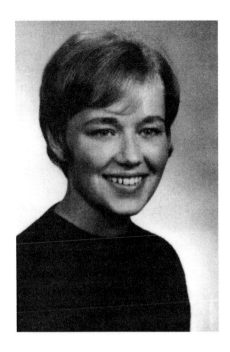

Diane Lindstrom of Rockford, Illinois. The high school student chose to forego a leg amputation in favor of taking Krebiozen for her bone cancer.

to walk around and do simple gardening once again. He literally came back to life."[30]

Friedman became chair of a group called Cancer Survivors on Krebiozen and led a vigorous lobbying effort on behalf of the drug. The group's biggest concern was the government's threat to ban interstate shipment of Krebiozen unless Ivy and Durovic complied with the new federal drug laws by filing a new plan by June 7, 1963, for continuing experimental use of the medicine. The plan would have to include much more comprehensive information about Krebiozen than the drug's sponsors had provided to that point. Friedman viewed Ivy and Durovic as "the men who saved my husband's life," and she placed all the responsibility for the impending ban on the government: "Someone is going to answer to me if they cut off this drug to the thousands of Krebiozen users."[31]

Friedman began a letter-writing campaign to recruit people to travel to Washington, DC, in May. A dozen members of Congress gathered in the Caucus Room of the Old Senate Office Building at the invitation of Senator Paul Douglas, and they listened as some fifty supporters of Krebiozen made an emotional appeal for the drug. Friedman introduced her somber and frail-looking husband, George. "I'm not one of the best cases, but I am still with you," he told the gathering. Additional testimonials from other patients followed. The next day, a larger contingent of more than one hundred Krebiozen supporters converged on the auditorium of the

Department of Health, Education, and Welfare. Boisfeuillet Jones was the only HEW official present. The patients and family members repeated their demands that interstate shipment of the drug not be halted, to little apparent effect. "We were dismayed but not surprised by the concern of the F.D.A. and H.E.W. with the legalisms rather than whether or not we lived or died," Friedman reported afterward.[32]

With the June 7 deadline only days away, Friedman's group returned to Washington and picketed the White House. A picture of Friedman being arrested appeared in the *Washington Post*. She had been accused of blocking the sidewalk while carrying a sign reading "Mr. President—Save Our Lives—Stop the Ban on Krebiozen." After paying ten dollars bond, she was released. The picketers managed to capture the attention of Dr. Peter Bing, a medical adviser to President Kennedy. Bing arranged a meeting with Ivy, Durovic, and HEW's Jones, and afterward it was announced that Ivy and Durovic had submitted their new plan for experimental use of Krebiozen, apparently preserving access to the drug.[33]

Any sense of triumph among the pro-Krebiozen contingent was shortlived. On July 12, Durovic abruptly withdrew the plan for continuing the

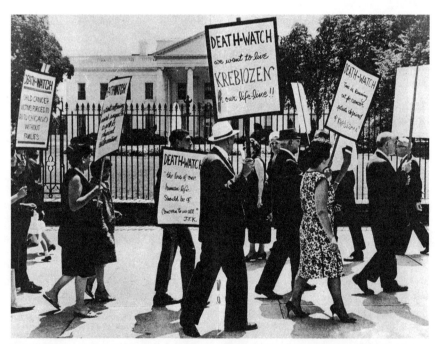

Pro-Krebiozen picketers outside the White House in August 1963. This photo was included in a pamphlet circulated by the drug's supporters. (Harry Ransom Center, The University of Texas at Austin)

use of the medicine, meaning that Krebiozen was now legally available only in Illinois, where it was manufactured. Friedman's group responded by returning to Washington once more in August. This time, more than two hundred black-clad picketers staged what they called a "death watch" in front of the White House and HEW's offices. They bore signs saying such things as "Cancer Patients Killed by Regulation." Friedman said that her husband had temporarily moved to Chicago so that he could continue to receive Krebiozen. "Cutting our Krebiozen lifeline is condemning many of us to a few weeks or months of intense suffering, to be followed by the finality of death," she said. William Pack of Brooklyn, New York, joined the picketers, saying that his ten-year-old son suffered from leukemia. "Eighteen months ago the doctors gave him little hope of living much longer," said Pack. "Against their advice we gave him Krebiozen. Two weeks ago he pitched a no-hit ball game. Now . . ." Pack could speak no more, and he began to weep.[34]

The interstate ban on Krebiozen remained in place. A few days after Friedman's latest trip to Washington, her husband George died. Pathologists who reviewed lab specimens of his cancer said that he had suffered from a "lazy tumor," a condition with which a person could live for years. His tumor type seemed to be the reason why he had survived for as long as he had—not Krebiozen. The previous January, Freda DeKnight also had died. She had maintained her faith in Ivy and Durovic's drug, and her family requested that donations in her memory be sent to the Krebiozen Research Foundation. One of her friends, though, suggested that her work had been what really sustained her: "Without the Fashion Fair to worry about, Freda would have gone long ago."[35]

In May 1963, only weeks after Diane Lindstrom had garnered widespread publicity for her decision to use Krebiozen, it was reported that she had abandoned the drug. According to her father, she had been experiencing pain and had fallen in the clinic where she had been receiving Krebiozen injections. An examination found that her "tumor had broken open." Lindstrom and her parents then flew to Raymondville, Texas, where eighty-two-year-old Isaac Newton Frost operated a clinic and administered a vaccine that he claimed cured cancer. "We're putting ourselves in his hands," Lindstrom's father said. After three months of treatments with no positive results, Lindstrom and her parents left Texas. She returned to her hometown of Rockford, Illinois, and entered a hospital. In late October, she died, conscious almost to the end, with her parents at her side.[36]

As for Rachel Carson, her experiment with Krebiozen did not last long. She had begun taking the drug in April 1963. "Krebiozen is still a hope, but only that," she wrote to Dorothy Freeman in May. In July, she stopped the medicine, having received no pain relief or any other benefit. Carson spent a final summer in her cottage in Southport, Maine, near the sea that she loved and had worked so hard to conserve. Freeman's granddaughter recalled one occasion when Carson was too ill to walk to the beach: "We all still had a lovely summer day going down and bringing little creatures up to the cottage for her to look at, and talk to us about, and then instruct us that they had to go back where they came from." Carson's health continued to decline, and she died the following spring.[37]

• • •

The conflict between the government and Ivy and Durovic over the new plan for experimental use of Krebiozen had been the culmination of months of sniping between the two sides. In response to the government's announcement in January 1963 that it was launching an investigation of the drug, Ivy and Durovic proposed bringing "a large number of cancer patients, who have responded very well to treatment with Krebiozen, for presentation to your medical staff in Washington." HEW's Boisfeuillet Jones responded that "the presentation of patients to give testimonials without any opportunity for prior study of their complete medical records would contribute nothing at all toward solution of the scientific question of Krebiozen's merit as an anti-cancer drug." To the public, HEW reiterated what the government actually required: reliable information about how the drug was made, proof of its safety, and convincing evidence that it actually might help treat cancer. According to HEW, the "basic difficulty is that Drs. Ivy and Durovic either cannot or will not supply this necessary information."[38]

Gilbert Goldhammer, head of the FDA Division of Regulatory Management, was directing the Krebiozen investigation. He and Kenneth Milstead of the agency's Bureau of Enforcement assigned Robert Palmer to the investigation. Palmer's previous work for the FDA had included going undercover as a truck driver to break up an illegal amphetamine ring; that operation had been dramatized in the Hollywood movie *Death in Small Doses*. Palmer also had helped terminate a promotional scheme for a device called a Spectro-Chrome, which supposedly fought disease by using lights and glass slides to coordinate with magnetic waves and ocean tides. Palmer now joined fellow FDA investigators Roland Sherman and Robert Scheno in trying to uncover the details about Krebiozen's manufacture and distribution that Ivy and Durovic were not providing.[39]

According to one observer, the FDA—although performing a critically important and indispensable function—never has managed to cultivate an image of congeniality. On the contrary, its staff members have often been viewed as "bureaucratic, unlikeable, stick-in-the-mud science addicts" dedicated to "hunting down scofflaws and chewing them up like Flintstone vitamins."[40] So it would be with the FDA and Krebiozen. Investigators tried doggedly to pin down the drug's sponsors, but they would find it frustratingly difficult to achieve their goal, and some of the tactics that they employed would do nothing to enhance their popularity.

In February 1963, the investigators visited Promak Laboratories in Chicago for the first time. Promak was the name that Durovic had given to the company that produced Krebiozen; its offices were located a few blocks south of Ivy's Roosevelt University laboratory. The investigators' first goal was to copy case histories of patients treated with Krebiozen—histories that the government believed were essential in determining what effects, if any, the drug was having on the people who took it. From the start, the investigators encountered resistance from Durovic, who, at one point, insisted that they had done enough copying. Nonetheless, they continued with the slow and tedious work, using a photo laboratory to transfer the records to microfilm. By the start of May, they had copied 508 sets of records.[41]

Those records represented what Ivy and Durovic said were the best and most complete case histories from among the more than four thousand people who had used Krebiozen. The FDA still considered the records to be inadequate. It began amassing additional information for each patient, including lab reports, X-rays, pathology slides, and, in some cases, death certificates and autopsy reports. The FDA directly contacted patients and their families for the information. In one such instance, the agency wrote to a man whose wife had recently died. "We realize that a discussion of her case is difficult for you," the FDA told him, while still expressing hope that he "would furnish us with signed releases so that medical records of the case may be obtained from the various other physicians and the hospitals concerned. We have enclosed several such forms and a self-addressed envelope for your convenience." FDA representatives even visited the homes of dying people to ask them and their family members to sign affidavits. In addition, the FDA checked the status of people who Ivy and Durovic claimed had been restored to health by Krebiozen. For instance, they had reported that Leonardo Taietti, a member of the Argentinian consulate in Chicago, was "well and free of complaints now" thanks to Krebiozen. In actuality, Taietti had died of cancer in Argentina several years previously.[42]

After finishing copying patient records, representatives of the FDA and the National Institutes of Health proceeded with field inspections of Krebiozen's production procedures. They went to Rockford, Illinois, to visit the Quaker Oats plant that manufactured Ken-L Ration dog food. Advertisements for Ken-L Ration featured a memorable jingle ("my dog's better than your dog!"); as of 1963, they also included a declaration that the food was made from "U.S. Gov't Inspected Horsemeat." According to Durovic, the dog food plant was where he administered the *Actinomyces bovis* bacterium to horses and then drew the blood used to create Krebiozen. The government representatives interviewed several Quaker Oats officials and a private veterinarian who worked for Durovic, but they found scant documentation of what precisely was happening at the plant in the production of Krebiozen. They also failed to obtain a sample of the horse plasma. Durovic, knowing that FDA investigators wanted to inspect the plasma, thwarted them by calling the Rockford plant and asking it to send him the remaining blood supply immediately. He then told the investigators that he had found the blood to be spoiled, so he poured it all down the drain.[43]

Robert Palmer and his FDA colleagues persisted in trying to uncover evidence of how Krebiozen was made by attempting to review purchase records of the supplies used to manufacture the drug. "Dr. Durovic told me there was only one trouble, and that was he didn't know where these records were," Palmer would recall. "He said that as a European he was accustomed to dealing with cash out of his pocket instead of writing checks." Palmer also received an odd message relayed by one of Durovic's lawyers, James Griffin. The message warned the FBI investigator of a "Kurse of Krebiozen" and added that "everybody who approached Krebiozen with malice has met with misfortune."[44]

Unbowed, Palmer told Durovic that he wanted to witness firsthand the production of the drug. What the FDA investigators had seen so far of the Promak laboratory made them highly suspicious that Durovic was creating the medicine in the exact manner that he had claimed. For instance, he had said that he used ethyl ether to separate Krebiozen powder from the horse plasma. However, the room at Promak in which that process was said to occur had no ventilation other than sash windows opening to the street, suggesting that the ether fumes would have been overpowering if not asphyxiating. Durovic tried to allay the FDA's suspicions by saying that he had switched from ethyl ether to benzene, but the FDA could find no company within three hundred miles of Chicago that had ever sold him benzene.[45]

On June 5, while Durovic and Ivy were in Washington, DC, Palmer told Durovic via telephone that he and his fellow investigators were prepared to visit Promak daily until they saw Krebiozen being made. "My God, don't do it," Durovic exclaimed. He told Palmer to wait until he returned to Chicago, which might not be for some time. Palmer and Roland Sherman responded by staking out Promak. Just three days later, on Saturday, June 8, they saw Durovic enter the laboratory. The FDA investigators followed him inside, and a bizarre and protracted confrontation ensued. "You want to see manufacturing operations? I'm going to show you manufacturing operations," Durovic said. He poured what he said was Krebiozen mixed in mineral oil into a bottle labeled as containing distilled water. Palmer told Durovic that it was not good practice to put drugs in improperly labeled containers, and Sherman photographed the bottle. Durovic erupted: "This is a frame-up!" He insisted that the FDA would use the photo to make it look as though Krebiozen was nothing but distilled water. Multiple telephone calls followed, with Durovic calling his attorneys and Palmer withdrawing to a public phone booth to call the FDA's Kenneth Milstead and William Goodrich in Washington. Goodrich, who was the agency's chief legal officer, was paged from the golf course. He urged Palmer to stand firm. Finally, over Durovic's protests, Palmer obtained samples of the Krebiozen-mineral oil solution, but he could not get any Krebiozen powder undissolved in the oil.[46]

There were more fraught encounters and angry phone calls over the next several days. Palmer and Sherman visited a former Chicago fire station where they had heard that Krebiozen was being put in ampules. They were confronted by Durovic's brother Marko, who said that the government was "conducting itself in a disgraceful and persecuting manner." Attorney Griffin told Palmer on the phone that he was disgusted with the FDA. "He asked if I had ever seen a drug product prepared under better conditions with better equipment and in a nicer laboratory," Palmer reported. "I told Mr. Griffin that I could not answer that question because I had never seen Krebiozen manufactured. Mr. Griffin blew up at this." Claiming government harassment, Durovic sued HEW Secretary Anthony Celebreeze in late June, but Judge Julius Hoffman in Chicago refused to issue a temporary injunction to halt the FDA investigation, and the suit eventually was dismissed. On July 12, Palmer at last succeeded in procuring a tiny sample of Krebiozen powder. Yet on that same day, Durovic wrote to Celebreeze to inform him that he was withdrawing the plan for continuing experimental use of Krebiozen. "I was subjected to abuses by your agents. They even made in my Laboratory a fraudulent photograph in order to smear me," Durovic wrote. "Under these circumstances you will understand, sir, that I have lost hope that your Department will ever solve this controversy in good faith." HEW's Boisfeuillet Jones replied to Durovic that the government denied all of his accusations while reminding him that interstate shipment of Krebiozen was now illegal.[47]

Although the FDA had failed to observe Krebiozen being produced, its investigators had seen enough to bolster the government's case against the drug. Palmer estimated that Promak held some five thousand glass ampules at a time when Durovic said that he had only enough Krebiozen to fill a few hundred ampules at most. It seemed as though the excess ampules were being filled by something else that was claimed to be the drug. Durovic also had said that it was extraordinarily expensive to manufacture the medicine; at one point, he had offered to sell the government a bit of Krebiozen powder for $170,000 per gram. He had claimed that he had to ask for nine dollars and fifty cents per ampule to recover his costs, adding that Krebiozen was being distributed for free to at least two-thirds of the people who requested it. Palmer and his colleagues learned that in fact 85 to 90 percent of people were paying for the drug. Moreover, the FDA had meticulously calculated the true manufacturing expenses of Krebiozen. Rather than costing almost ten dollars to produce a single ampule, the actual cost was only eight cents.[48]

The FDA was also investigating where the drug was being shipped. The agency already had sent phony letters to the Krebiozen Research Foundation, supposedly from patients who wanted Krebiozen after having undergone such drastic operations as the removal of both their lungs. That such procedures would have been obviously fatal to the "patients" seemed not to matter to the foundation, which had offered to send the drug in return for cash donations. Now, with interstate shipment of Krebiozen having been banned, the FDA began surveillance of both Promak's offices and Ivy's laboratory, looking for out-of-state license plates indicating that people were traveling to Chicago to acquire the drug and then illegally transporting it out of Illinois. (The interstate ban, on top of doctors' increasing reluctance to get Krebiozen for their patients, had heightened people's worries about accessing the medicine; in one instance, a woman broke into Promak with a hammer, screwdriver, and glass cutter to steal the drug.) In addition, the FDA placed an investigator with a plastic bag on Chicago sanitation trucks that were picking up garbage from the offices of Krebiozen's sponsors. "When they dumped the garbage, we had them dump it into the plastic bag," one investigator remembered, adding that they then would sift through the garbage to garner information on out-of-state patients. In the case of Krebiozen proponent Dr. William Phillips, FDA representatives personally raided his garbage can in the middle of the night, heedless of concerns that they might be trespassing.[49]

The biggest breakthrough in the investigation of Krebiozen, though, would happen hundreds of miles from Chicago, inside the FDA's laboratories in the Washington, DC, area. Frank Wiley, the director of the FDA's Division of Pharmaceutical Chemistry, was trying at long last to determine what Krebiozen was. He had nothing to work with except purported samples of the medicine mixed in mineral oil, plus three infrared spectrograms of the drug. When it proved impossible to extract Krebiozen powder from the oil, the spectrograms were the only remaining clues. Wiley turned to analytical chemist Alma LeVant Hayden. She had attended a historically Black university, South Carolina State College, with plans of becoming a nurse. "I got so interested in chemistry that I gave up that idea," she recalled. Instead, after earning a graduate degree at Howard University, she joined the FDA in 1956, likely becoming the first African American woman scientist there. For years, the FDA had refused to hire Black scientists. The rationale, according to an FDA official in 1946, was that the agency's scientists "occasionally have to appear in court to support a case or offer testimony on findings. A colored person might prejudice the case in court in certain sections of the country."[50]

Soon after the FDA launched its Krebiozen investigation in 1963, Hayden was named head of the agency's spectrophotometry branch because of her expertise in using cutting-edge techniques to identify chemical substances. Spectrophotometry measured the wavelengths of light absorbed by a substance, and it produced a graph—a spectrogram—of the substance's chemical fingerprint. Hayden's FDA team began sifting through a catalog containing twenty thousand spectrograms of known compounds, trying

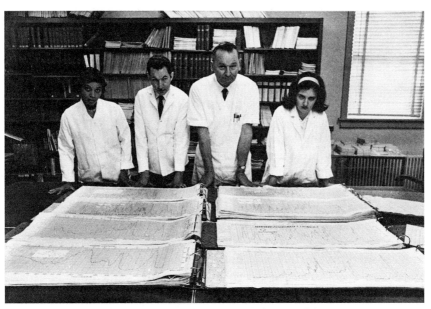

Members of the FDA team that discovered that Krebiozen was creatine (from left to right): Alma LeVant Hayden, Wilson Brannon, Oscar Sammul, and Ruth Kessler. (Courtesy of the Food and Drug Administration)

to find a match with the three Krebiozen spectrograms. "As a diversion, we discussed why ancient civilizations sprang up where they did," team member Oscar Sammul remembered. "We had to take little breaks. After all, it was pretty monotonous work." Even so, only a few hours after they had begun their search, Ruth Kessler—a twenty-year-old University of Pennsylvania chemistry major and FDA summer assistant—made a startling discovery. The Krebiozen spectrograms were virtually identical to a spectrogram of creatine, a compound widely present in the human body. Hayden and the other team members confirmed Kessler's findings.[51]

The FDA was determined to clinch its case "frontwards and backwards," as one of its officials later put it. The agency formed four new teams consisting of both FDA scientists and outside scientists; one of the teams was headed by Hayden. Each team used a different scientific technique to analyze part of the miniscule specimen of Krebiozen powder that Robert Palmer had labored so mightily to obtain from Ivy and Durovic in July. In each instance, the powder was found to be creatine or a breakdown product called creatinine. The FDA took extraordinary pains to ensure that there were multiple witnesses to each step of the analytical process in order to rebut potential charges that the agency had tested something other than the specimen that Ivy and Durovic had provided. The agency also examined ampules of Krebiozen that had been shipped in the past; they were discovered to contain nothing but mineral oil, just as two California experts had testified back in 1958.[52]

The FDA announced its findings in early September 1963. T. Phillip Waalkes, chief of the NCI's chemotherapy program, noted that creatine had shown no effect on cancer in animals. As for using it as an anticancer agent in humans, Waalkes said that "it would be impossible to conceive that Krebiozen in the doses used would have any value in view of the large amounts" of creatine already in the body. Each day the average person produced one hundred thousand times the amount of creatine found in a Krebiozen ampule. It also was noted that creatine could be easily extracted from hamburger meat and purchased from chemical supply houses for only thirty cents a gram, vastly less than what Durovic had been asking for Krebiozen.[53]

A reporter contacted George Stoddard, who was now serving as chancellor of New York University. Eleven years previously, while still president of the University of Illinois, Stoddard had declared that if Krebiozen existed at all, it was nothing more than a harmless, common substance. When the news came that he finally had been shown to be correct, friends brought champagne to his house to drink a celebratory toast. To the reporter, Stoddard expressed sympathy for the people with cancer who had used

Krebiozen instead of a therapy that actually worked. He did express one note of self-satisfaction: "One doesn't have to be a scientist, but only an experienced administrator, to smell a rat."[54]

At the same time that the FDA was declaring that it had found Krebiozen to be creatine, the NCI was completing a review of the more than five hundred patient case histories that the FDA had copied at the offices of Krebiozen's sponsors. NCI director Kenneth Endicott convened a blue-ribbon committee to study the histories and determine whether they justified the clinical test of Krebiozen that the drug's supporters had been calling for all along. The twenty-four committee members came from all over the country and were experienced in every facet of diagnosing and treating cancer, including surgery, radiotherapy, chemotherapy, internal medicine, pathology, and endocrinology. Because many of the histories were of breast cancer patients, several doctors with expertise in that area were included on the committee. In August, the committee members were sequestered in a motel in Bethesda, Maryland, and they began examining the patient records.[55]

The committee issued its report in October. It rejected the idea that such subjective data as patient reports of pain relief and well-being showed that Krebiozen worked. "The use of subjective response in evaluating the effectiveness of an agent without reference to objective regression [of tumors] is treacherous," the committee said. "The administration of any new agent almost invariably improves the patient's outlook and hope for some period of time." The committee instead reviewed whatever objective data it could derive from the case histories. More than two hundred cases were deemed "inadequate test situations"; the patients had received conventional therapies in addition to Krebiozen, or else they never had been diagnosed with cancer or had shown no trace of cancer when they started taking the drug. As for the remaining 288 cases, 273 showed no objective benefit from Krebiozen. Thirteen cases showed equivocal results, with "questions concerning the actual amount of decrease in tumor size, the true validity of the measurements or statements given, and the precise status of the disease. Inadequate documentation often made accurate assessment difficult." That left only two cases—out of the more than five hundred cases that the NCI had analyzed—in which Krebiozen seemed to be associated with objective improvements in patients, a minute percentage that the committee said might be found in any large, random sample of people with cancer who had been treated with an unproven substance. "It is the unanimous opinion of the Review Committee that Krebiozen is ineffective as an antitumor agent," the report concluded.[56]

Endicott followed up the NCI committee's report with his own statement on Krebiozen. He said that a clinical trial of any drug would have to be justified on one of three bases, none of which Krebiozen met. The first basis was theoretical: "The proponents of 'Krebiozen' have advanced the theory that 'Krebiozen' is a tissue hormone which inhibits the multiplication of cancer cells. The Food and Drug Administration has demonstrated that 'Krebiozen' is not a tissue hormone but rather creatine, a normal component of the human body concerned primarily with muscle contraction." The second basis for a clinical trial was animal testing, and Krebiozen's proponents never had submitted reliable data showing that the drug had antitumor effects in animals. The third basis was the "accidental discovery that a drug has anticancer activity in human beings," and the NCI review committee had just reported its conviction that Krebiozen was ineffective in that regard. Therefore, said Endicott, there was "no justification for a clinical trial" of the drug, "and from a scientific standpoint we regard the case closed."[57]

The FDA and the NCI had delivered a staggering double blow to Krebiozen. The agencies had officially pronounced the drug worthless while declaring that a government test of the medicine would never happen. What was more, it appeared increasingly likely that Ivy and the Durovic brothers would face criminal charges. "With the facts that have been reported to us by our investigators," FDA Commissioner George Larrick announced, "the normal course would be to recommend that these people be given an opportunity to show cause why they should not be prosecuted in federal court."[58]

Larrick was not necessarily eager to press the legal case against Krebiozen. He had garnered a reputation for being soft on the pharmaceutical industry in its dealings with the FDA, and when it came to prosecuting quackery, he already had seen the FDA fail twice to win a jury verdict against William Frederick Koch's Glyoxylide cancer treatment. In 1960, Larrick had told the *New York Post* that he "would hate like the devil" to try to contest Krebiozen in a similar jury trial.[59] Krebiozen's proponents would immediately make it clear that they would not submit meekly to the government's dismissal of the drug. The medicine's biggest supporter in Congress was about to submit a report of his own—one based on his own independent research—and he would mount one last push for a government test of Krebiozen, this time with the personal backing of the president of the United States.

CHAPTER 6

The Emperor's New Clothes

Paul Douglas had always been a maverick. As a young economics professor at the University of Chicago in the 1920s, he espoused socialism during a markedly laissez-faire era. After he was elected to the Chicago City Council in 1939, he vexed the Kelly-Nash machine that had backed his candidacy by frequently bucking the machine's political positions. When the machine derailed his candidacy for a US Senate seat in 1942, Douglas joined the US Marines at age fifty during World War II. He talked his way into combat in the Pacific and was awarded a Bronze Star and two Purple Hearts for wounds that cost him partial use of his left arm. After a lengthy hospital stay, Douglas returned to Illinois, ran again for the Senate as a Democrat in 1948, and won handily. *Time* magazine devoted a cover story to him two years later, describing him as "a rumpled, craggy, mountain of a man" and "a liberal who has learned a healthy skepticism of the liberal cliches." Over time—when reelected in 1954 and 1960—Douglas came to be known as the "conscience of the Senate."[1]

Even Douglas's supporters acknowledged that he had his foibles. "Douglas's piety and ingenuousness, though generally regarded as enviable, left him open to charges of superciliousness," his biographer would write. One of his fellow senators once crossly asked him if he viewed himself as Jesus Christ. Although Douglas championed civil rights and other liberal causes, some of his pet initiatives seemed quixotic. He lobbied for a new kind of bread that he insisted was more nutritious than what was being offered commercially; he also lobbied on behalf of a type of fish flour. As a result, he would acknowledge that he earned a reputation as a "food faddist." Douglas also tangled with the Food and Drug Administration, which he said exemplified "bureaucracy and the insolence of office" through its refusal to

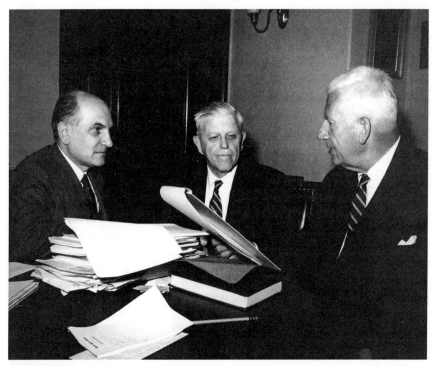

Stevan Durovic (left) and Andrew Ivy (center) with US Senator Paul Douglas of Illinois (right). Douglas asked President Lyndon B. Johnson to help arrange a test of Krebiozen in 1964. (Courtesy of the University of Illinois at Urbana-Champaign Archives, image 0012175)

allow such food products to reach the market. The senator's opinion of the American Medical Association, the implacable opponent of public health insurance, was no better than his estimation of the FDA.[2]

Douglas's embrace of Krebiozen was therefore not out of character for him, particularly in light of his decades-long friendship with Andrew Ivy, whom he had first met at the University of Chicago. Douglas had steadfastly backed Ivy's call for a so-called fair test of Krebiozen despite the AMA's rejection of the drug. When the National Cancer Institute had resisted testing the medicine, Douglas had gone so far as to challenge the NCI's funding. Now, even though both the NCI and the FDA had publicly repudiated Krebiozen, Douglas still would not be dissuaded from supporting the medicine. According to his biographer, Douglas held a "lifelong attraction to the cause of the underdog," and no one seemed more of an underdog than Ivy.[3]

Ivy's own faith in Krebiozen remained unshaken. After the FDA reported that it had found the drug to be creatine, Ivy branded the report as "ridiculous, apparently a fraud, and a smear"—precisely what he had done in attacking similar negative assessments of the drug in the past. Krebiozen was soluble in mineral oil whereas creatine was not, Ivy said. Stevan Durovic responded to the FDA report by writing again to Anthony Celebreeze at the Department of Health, Education, and Welfare. Durovic claimed that his own chemists had found Krebiozen to have a molecular weight greater than that of creatine and to have a different chemical composition as well. "I cannot refrain from calling your attention to the predicament of those patients in whom it has been shown that 'Krebiozen' is necessary for the maintenance of their health and life," Durovic wrote. "Who is going to assume the moral responsibility for the care of these patients?" Some of those patients and their family members attended a news conference that Ivy and Durovic held in New York. "It is not Krebiozen that is on the spot," cried Alexander Gabriel, a radio journalist whose wife had used the drug. "It is the American conscience and the morality of the American government that is at stake!"[4]

Government officials and much of the press had wearied of the protestations of the Krebiozen supporters. HEW's Boisfeuillet Jones replied to Durovic's letter with a point-by-point defense of the FDA's findings, which Jones called "scientifically unimpeachable" in proving beyond doubt that Krebiozen was creatine. Regarding Durovic's ominous warnings about the future health of Krebiozen patients, Jones was blunt: "You and Dr. Ivy have encouraged their belief; you made 'Krebiozen' available to them with claims of benefit. . . . The full moral responsibility for the consequence is yours." As for the press, *Chicago Daily News* science writer Arthur Snider reported that although about two hundred journalists showed up for the start of another news conference that Ivy held in Washington after the FDA's and NCI's negative assessments of Krebiozen, the reporters soon began to walk out, and only a few remained by the end of the event. Snider called it a "saddening valedictory" for Ivy, who once had been "a fountainhead of press information on important advances in medicine." Even Boston newspaper columnist George Frazier—the author of multiple articles blasting Krebiozen's opponents—had grown disillusioned. "At this point, the dispassionate evidence against Ivy and Durovic is overwhelming. I'm very unhappy," Frazier wrote to Senator Douglas's chief aide Howard Shuman.[5]

Shuman was fiercely devoted to Douglas, as were the rest of the senator's aides. "We took a ride on his magic carpet," Shuman would fondly recall of the senator, adding that "those who worked for him probably experienced the greatest public moments in their lives." Shuman emphatically agreed with Douglas that Krebiozen was not being treated fairly by the US government; the senator's aide always would believe that the drug as originally formulated by Durovic had worked every bit as well as Ivy had claimed back in 1951. Shuman helped form a four-person independent research group to examine the government's evidence against Krebiozen. Apart from Shuman himself, the group included Illinois scientists Scott Anderson and Howard Clark, with Dr. Miles Robinson of Potomac, Maryland, serving as chair. Anderson and Clark each held strong research credentials, and each man operated his own laboratory in Champaign-Urbana. Robinson, described by one reporter as being "independently well-off and independent-minded," had previously chaired a conference of the National Health Federation, an organization that boosted nonmainstream medicine and opposed vaccine mandates. According to Robinson, the FDA was "in the hip pocket of the A.M.A, which in turn is heavily under the influence of the drug companies." He was convinced that the government was "absolutely wrong" in its assessment of Krebiozen.[6]

Douglas's group submitted its report to the senator at the start of December 1963, and Douglas immediately took to the Senate floor to deliver a lengthy, impassioned defense of Krebiozen. His office would republish his remarks under the heading "FDA Mistaken, Krebiozen Not Creatine: NCI Judgment of Cases Biased and Irrelevant: Evidence Justifies Fair Test Now." Douglas rejected virtually everything that the government had amassed against the drug, including the FDA's analysis led by Alma LeVant Hayden and the NCI's analysis of more than five hundred patient case histories. Douglas pointed to studies by Anderson, who said that there were significant differences between the spectrograms of Krebiozen and those of creatine; the senator also cited studies by Clark, who said that Krebiozen contained sugars and acids that were not creatine. In fact, Krebiozen and creatine were not even the same color. Douglas charged that the NCI committee had "set extremely harsh and severe standards" in evaluating the case histories while refusing to meet with Ivy. "It is a terrible thing that we cannot really trust either the Food and Drug Administration or the National Cancer Institute," the senator added. He demanded that "neutral scientists" lead a new investigation of Krebiozen and that the FDA retract and apologize for its "false statements" about Ivy and Durovic.[7]

After publicly attacking the government's medical agencies, Douglas privately tried to arrange a test of Krebiozen by going straight to the top. In January 1964, the senator wrote to President Lyndon B. Johnson, who had just taken office upon John F. Kennedy's assassination. Douglas forwarded four letters from doctors who said that Krebiozen deserved a test, and he reiterated his fervent belief that Krebiozen was not creatine: "Mr. President, the Food and Drug Administration is *wrong*." The senator asked the president to set up a "distinguished committee in order to make some proper judgment about the drug's merits and potentialities." Soon afterward, Stevan Durovic approached Douglas and Shuman with what he said was good news—he had produced a new, purified batch of Krebiozen that was guaranteed to be creatine-free and that also was 50 percent more potent than any previous batch of the drug. Durovic said that he already had tested the new batch on a handful of patients with excellent results, and he had enough of it for tests on up to a hundred more patients.[8]

Fortified by Durovic's reassurances, Douglas pushed the case for Krebiozen during a face-to-face meeting with President Johnson in March. Johnson had responded to the senator's initial letter by passing off the matter to HEW's Boisfeuillet Jones, who already had made clear his low opinion of the drug. Douglas wanted the president to form the hoped-for evaluation committee without Jones's participation. The senator and the president had had a long and often testy relationship. While Senate majority leader in the 1950s, Johnson on occasion had treated Douglas badly, and Douglas had mistrusted Johnson. As president, though, Johnson would advance many of the liberal domestic initiatives that Douglas held dear, including the Civil Rights Act of 1964 and the Voting Rights Act of 1965; in turn, Douglas would staunchly support Johnson's hawkish policy toward Vietnam. The president chose to accede to Douglas's entreaties on behalf of Krebiozen, directing White House aide Myer Feldman to help set up the committee that the senator wanted.[9]

Subsequent negotiations over the committee took place largely between Douglas's office and the office of presidential science adviser Donald Hornig. At one point, the negotiations hit a snag. "We were informed that there is dramatic new evidence on the purification of Krebiozen and on its efficacy in a limited number of patients with cancer," Hornig wrote to Douglas in early April. "What concerns me, however, is that to date no information on the new preparation or its effectiveness has been provided to us." Douglas responded with "considerable amazement" that Hornig seemed adamant about receiving such information before allowing the committee's work to proceed. Hornig did not press the point, and both sides agreed to the committee's members: doctors Frank Adair, Wallace Graham, William McElroy, and Richard Shope. Adair and Graham were among the doctors whose testimonials for Krebiozen had already been forwarded by Douglas to the president, while McElroy and Shope were the White House's choices for the committee.[10]

Douglas's correspondence with Hornig suggested that the senator had complete faith that Durovic would soon deliver the corroborating evidence about his new batch of Krebiozen. A frequent criticism of Durovic was that his furtiveness about the drug made it impossible to determine whether one batch of the medicine was the same as another. In Douglas's Senate speech, he acknowledged that there had been different formulations of Krebiozen over the years and that some of them had contained creatine. Nonetheless, said Douglas, each formulation was at heart the same drug, and Krebiozen was not now and never had been solely creatine as the FDA had charged. The senator also entered into the Congressional Record letters that Abbott Laboratories and Eli Lilly had sent to Durovic in 1951 expressing interest in marketing Krebiozen. Douglas said that Durovic had turned down the pharmaceutical companies' overtures for fear that they would charge too much for the drug. The senator soon received an angry letter from Eli Lilly saying that he should have known that Durovic had "consistently refused to reveal the processes for producing krebiozen and sought to operate in an atmosphere of secrecy wholly foreign to science and to American medicine." The company added that it resented Douglas's implication that it had "intended to profiteer at the expense of cancer victims."[11]

Despite his public expressions of support, Douglas had held his own skepticism toward Durovic virtually from the start, telling him back in 1951 that had Ivy not personally endorsed Durovic's drug, "I would be very skeptical of the whole damn thing."[12] Other Krebiozen supporters were now making their frustrations public. Ivy's attorney, John Sembower, said that Durovic's abrupt decision in July 1963 to withdraw the plan for continuing experimental use of Krebiozen was "typical of Durovic's singlemindedness and monomania." Even Ivy was said to be "steamed" over Durovic's unilateral action, which had made interstate shipment of the drug illegal.[13] Ivy would tell Howard Shuman and Miles Robinson that the Yugoslavian doctor had embarrassed him on two other occasions: when Durovic had dissolved all the original Krebiozen powder in mineral oil, and more recently when Durovic had given the FDA a Krebiozen sample that turned out to be mostly creatine (even though Ivy remained adamant that it was not 100 percent creatine).[14]

Douglas's office decided to lay down strict criteria that Durovic and Ivy would have to fulfill before they would be allowed to meet with the new evaluation committee that the senator had fought so hard to set up. "I have put my head on the block for you," Douglas told the two men via telegram in late April 1964. He said that they needed to submit a sample of the new, purified batch of Krebiozen for analysis at a Chicago lab and also at Howard Clark's and Scott Anderson's labs in Champaign-Urbana. They needed to explain the production process for Krebiozen "much more thoroughly than you have done so far so that when we go before the committee there will be no questions about this." They needed to test the new batch on at least ten breast cancer patients and produce photographs showing that improvements in the patients' conditions were directly attributable to the drug. They also needed to have enough Krebiozen powder on hand to proceed with tests on additional patients. "All this is crucial," Douglas told Ivy and Durovic. "We are up against the gun. You must make good. This is the last real chance."[15]

Had Durovic been telling the truth about the good results already achieved with the new Krebiozen, there should have been little difficulty in meeting Douglas's conditions and proceeding with a scheduled meeting with the committee on June 1. Almost immediately, though, Durovic began exhibiting a familiar pattern of delay and obfuscation. When Shuman pressed him during a phone conversation in early May, Durovic hedged on when lab tests of the drug might be available, and he accused Shuman of showing no confidence in him. Durovic also ignored multiple entreaties to deliver information about the purified Krebiozen's manufacture or chemistry. Miles Robinson traveled twice to Chicago to check on the small group of patients who Durovic said had benefitted from the new batch of the drug. One patient responded just as well to a placebo as she had to Krebiozen, and Durovic had given incorrect information about another patient's cancer. Douglas's office repeated its insistence that Durovic "provide ten cases which could withstand the most ruthless criticism," but it received only half that number. In addition, Durovic kept delaying a visit to Washington that would allow the senator and his staff to review all of the information that they were supposed to receive prior to the June 1 meeting.[16]

Finally, on May 29, Durovic and Ivy arrived in Washington. Because of Durovic's previous procrastination, Douglas could not be present to meet with the two men, but he authorized Shuman to act on his behalf. Shuman quickly discovered to his "utter amazement" that "instead of a creatine-free Krebiozen," Durovic "had a new and different preparation composed of combinations of two or three well known chemicals." Durovic's other statements concerning the alleged new batch of the drug turned out to be false. There was not enough powder to conduct additional patient tests. Ivy told Shuman and Robinson that meeting the evaluation committee under such conditions would make them all look "ridiculous"; he also lamented that Durovic had embarrassed him yet again. Even so, Ivy still would not renounce either Durovic or Krebiozen.[17]

Shuman decided that he had no choice but to call Donald Hornig at the White House and call off the June 1 meeting. "The enormity of Dr. Ivy and Dr. Durovic's folly can perhaps be seen by this synopsis," Shuman wrote in a private memo a few days later. "The President of the United States agreed to set up a committee with at least two friendly members. This was done. We knew indirectly that both of these men were willing to go forward with a clinical test. The other two members had never been involved with the Krebiozen controversy, were men of unquestioned standing and gave every appearance of being fair minded." A positive assessment by the committee could have led to Ivy's scientific vindication and to renewed interstate distribution and even legal sale of the drug; it also could have forestalled federal indictments of Ivy and Durovic. Instead—over Durovic's vocal objections—the meeting with the committee was canceled. Shuman speculated that perhaps Ivy and Durovic had been unable to replicate the original Krebiozen; Ivy indicated that subsequent batches of the drug had been only one-fifth as potent as the initial batch (whereas Durovic had claimed that the latest batch was 50 percent *more* potent). Shuman also said that Durovic, "a terrific egoist," might have felt that he and Ivy could force a test of any concoction that they put before the committee. Either way, Shuman was disgusted with the two men: "They had a golden opportunity and they blew it. What folly!"[18]

Douglas told Ivy and Durovic how "extremely disappointed" he was in both of them, although he left the door open a crack if they ever managed to meet the criteria to which both sides had originally agreed. Durovic said that this might happen at an unspecified future date, but only if his "adversaries" allowed it. Douglas and Shuman never made public the extent to which Ivy and Durovic had betrayed their trust. To be sure, such a disclosure would have greatly embarrassed the senator, but Shuman also told Douglas that "it is hard to bring oneself to hit someone when they are already down." Indeed, as 1964 progressed, the prospects for Ivy and Durovic seemed increasingly bleak.[19]

• • •

Regardless of whatever else happened during this time, Krebiozen's supporters still rallied around the drug. Patients continued to travel to Illinois, the one place where they could legally obtain Krebiozen; Illinois attorney general William Clark had decided that the state could not ban it until after the federal government completed any legal action that it might take against the drug. Fifteen hundred people gathered in New York to demonstrate for Krebiozen and demand a congressional investigation of the FDA. Among the speakers were Allen Rutherford, the Pennsylvania doctor who was one of the drug's biggest backers; Laine Friedman, who had led picketing for Krebiozen outside the White House; and Herbert Bailey, author of the pro-Krebiozen manifesto *A Matter of Life or Death*. By 1964, Bailey had turned to other health-related causes, particularly the promotion of vitamin E. Nevertheless, he drew cheers at the New York demonstration when he called on NCI director Kenneth Endicott to resign because of Endicott's opposition to Krebiozen.[20]

If Bailey needed any additional motivation to speak at the demonstration, *A Matter of Life and Death* was about to be issued in paperback. Timex had contributed five thousand dollars toward its publication to help promote a new television documentary that the watch manufacturer was sponsoring.[21] The hour-long documentary was called *Krebiozen and Cancer: Thirteen Years of Bitter Controversy*, and it aired on seventy-five stations across the country at the end of May. As produced by David Wolper Productions and reported by Bill Stout, the program was scrupulously neutral, leaving viewers who otherwise had never heard of Krebiozen with little guidance on which side of the debate over the drug was more credible.[22] Opponents of the medicine did receive significant airtime; when the NCI's Endicott was asked what Krebiozen's sponsors had to do to get a government test of the medicine, he bluntly replied that they needed to "find a new drug that works." However, Ivy and Durovic were shown standing firmly behind Krebiozen while denying all the government's charges against it. A short montage depicted Durovic supposedly administering *Actinomyces bovis* to horses and then producing Krebiozen at Promak Laboratories in Chicago. Senator Douglas told Stout that the government already tested hundreds of other cancer remedies, some of them toxic, and therefore it ought to test Krebiozen as well; the senator also invoked previous pioneering doctors whose breakthroughs had been scorned by what he called "medical politicians." Pro-Krebiozen groups thought highly enough of the documentary to screen it at their meetings.[23]

The documentary included the story of nine-year-old Cathy Hodnett of New Jersey. In 1960, Cathy had been diagnosed with Wilms' tumor, a kidney cancer most often found in children. She underwent surgery and then radiation therapy, which triggered serious side effects. The radiation was stopped and Krebiozen was begun. Cathy's parents believed that the medicine was keeping their daughter cancer-free, and her father also would take it for his own cancer. Although her father died in 1963, Cathy remained on the drug, and she sent President Johnson a letter. "Dear Mr. President," she wrote, "I have a problem. My mother can't keep running back and forth from Chicago to get Krebiozen. I am glad you and your family are well, but there are many cancer patients who need Krebiozen. *I wish* you could do *something*." Pro-Krebiozen groups put Cathy's face on eighteen thousand postcards that were sent to the White House, and the groups also featured her image in flyers. "Cathy and all the other cancer patients using Krebiozen appeal to you," one flyer said. "The Nuremberg trials exposed the Nazis 'Crime against humanity' for injecting sick people, against their will, with a medication that killed them. Is it less a 'Crime against humanity' to withhold medication, against their will, from cancer patients who fear they will die without it"?[24]

Gertrude Brou of Florida was another such patient, having started Krebiozen in lieu of a radical mastectomy. In May 1964, Brou began a one-person picket of the White House that would last for more than a month, and she wrote her own letter to the president. "*I chose Krebiozen* not because I am terminal but because I had seen my sister in the worst agony of a cancer terminal patient which had started in the Breast," wrote Brou. "I *chose* Krebiozen because it made sense to me. A treatment which would help me the way insulin helps a diabetic." She believed that she should be allowed to use a medicine that did not hurt her and made her feel better. "The National Cancer Institute had 22 'experts' report Krebiozen ineffective in the treatment of cancer," Brou's letter continued. "Can I, living proof that Krebiozen or 'creatine' is effective, believe in these experts? Have they come up with a cure for cancer?" Brou was sentenced to ninety days in jail after picketing in a restricted area. She accused the government of cruel and unusual punishment by depriving her of Krebiozen while she was incarcerated. After her release, Brou moved to Chicago so that she could continue to access the drug, supporting herself by working in a coat-check room.[25]

Krebiozen supporters' efforts to move the government once again failed, while a number of journalists and academics weighed in against the medicine. The *Chicago Daily News* had by this point adopted a strongly anti-Krebiozen editorial position, and it pointed to the death of Diane Lindstrom (the Illinois teenager who had taken the drug instead of having her leg amputated) as a prime example of the evils of quackery. *Consumer Reports* commented that Paul Douglas's independent research group chaired by Miles Robinson had been "strangely staffed." The magazine added that its own medical consultants had found nothing that "invalidated or even affected the FDA conclusion as to Krebiozen's identity or the NCI's decision that no basis could be found to justify clinical tests." In the *Bulletin of Atomic Scientists*, Howard Margolis wrote that there was "no serious scientific content whatever" in the pro-Krebiozen arguments: "If Krebiozen should turn out to have any value, it would be quite as surprising as if it turned out that wearing a bag of salt around your neck would cure a cold."[26]

In October 1964, *Life* magazine published a devasting profile of Krebiozen's chief scientific proponent under the headline "What Ever Happened to Dr. Ivy?" After recounting Ivy's illustrious life and career up to 1951, the article detailed what it called the "tragic medical sideshow" of Krebiozen and the drug's "oddly assorted little band of fervid supporters." Ivy himself, now seventy-one years old, was described as old and shuffling, if still unbowed. One of his former students spoke of him sadly: "Here was a king of classroom and laboratory, a good and wise king, who surely had the capacity for solving the riddle of the Sphinx, but who in some unknowable way carried within his own greatness the seeds of his doom. You can see a tragic end coming toward him and you know it's inevitable. But you can't say when it will be." Incensed, Ivy sent a letter to *Life* challenging the article's author "to a boxing match at the nearest YMCA gymnasium or to a one-mile foot race in Grant Park, to occur the next time he comes to Chicago." Ivy also suggested that they go "to a psychiatrist and physiologist and ascertain who has the youngest mind and highest I.Q."[27]

Ivy's bluster could not mask the fact that he was facing criminal prosecution, just as the government had hinted would happen after the FDA identified Krebiozen as creatine. A grand jury convened in Chicago in October, and it returned indictments against four men: Ivy, Stevan and Marko Durovic, and Dr. William F. P. Phillips, the last of whom had been providing Krebiozen to patients for years. The Krebiozen Research Foundation also was named in the indictment. The defendants faced forty-nine counts of mail fraud, conspiracy, mislabeling, and making false statements to the government. The government charged that the Durovic brothers had deposited $3.7 million in their Chicago bank accounts, and they also had deposited $1.7 million in overseas accounts in Canada and Switzerland. Stevan Durovic claimed that the cash that had been taken out of the country had gone to repay people who had given him loans to develop Krebiozen: "That money was not mine. I am a poor man."[28]

Krebiozen users feared that the indictments might cut them off from the drug entirely. A group of about fifteen demonstrators held a sit-in at HEW's offices in Washington, calling once more for the government to stop suppressing the medicine. Among the demonstrators was Gertrude Brou, who was so distraught that a psychiatrist was called to assess her. Laine Friedman, another demonstrator, said that it was "inhuman" to make Brou suffer, and she added, "This is the bitter harvest, the tragedy we've been trying to avoid." Krebiozen supporters asked the United Nations to intervene and stop what they called a violation of their human rights, especially "the most sacred right of all—the right to live." A new lawsuit that Ivy filed to try to resume interstate shipment of the medicine failed.[29]

Ivy, the Durovic brothers, and Phillips all pleaded not guilty to the charges against them. "I'm willing to go to jail on the basis of my convictions," said Ivy. "I won't be the first scientist to be burned at the stake. Every step of progress has been by a good fanatic who at the time was thought to be a bad fanatic." San Francisco attorney George Davis was an unpaid legal consultant to Ivy. According to Davis, the upcoming trial raised the fundamental question of "whether a doctor, in his ethical and moral relationship to his client, can be denied the right to prescribe as he sees fit, and whether a patient who has been given up by orthodox medicine has a right to try medicine or therapy which in his opinion may either relieve his pain or otherwise help him." Davis said that he thought the trial would take about two months. It would end up lasting more than four times that long.[30]

• • •

The Krebiozen trial in federal district court in Chicago was overseen by Judge Julius Hoffman, who, back in July 1963, had refused to grant an injunction halting the FDA's investigation of Promak Laboratories. Hoffman already had acquired a decidedly mixed reputation. A diminutive man who often took a brisk two-mile walk from his Lake Shore Drive apartment to the federal courthouse in the Loop, Hoffman was noted for his erudition, work ethic, and wit, as well as his love of golf and ballroom dancing. Yet the judge also was known for having a big ego and a short fuse. He liked to be called "Julius the Just," and he delivered frequent tongue-lashings to attorneys, one of whom would describe him as "a sadistic old bastard." Hoffman's biggest notoriety would come a few years after the Krebiozen case, when he presided over the trial of the "Chicago Seven" antiwar protestors: a protracted spectacle whose highlights included the judge's order that one defendant be bound, gagged, and chained to a chair in the courtroom. The Krebiozen proceedings did not produce quite the same fireworks, but they were no less convoluted, and at times they mightily tried Hoffman's patience.[31]

Hoffman originally scheduled the Krebiozen trial to begin on January 11, 1965, but he soon postponed the proceedings in exasperation over what he called the defense's "highly technical" pretrial motions. "You asked me for a quick trial and I set an early date; now you wait to the last day to file motions," the judge exclaimed, accusing the defense of "misleading the court." At a subsequent hearing, Hoffman denied the defense motions, which had included moving the trial from Chicago because of negative publicity there about Krebiozen. "It seems to me naïve to think there is any section of the country where people do not have any interest in a drug that alleges to aid cancer victims," the judge said in rejecting the change of venue. As for the defense's charges of an "abuse of prosecutory responsibility," Hoffman retorted that he had never before heard the word "prosecutory." When Ivy slipped out of the courtroom during the hearing to meet with cancer patients, Hoffman ordered Ivy's lawyers to find and return him immediately: "I'll send a marshal for him if you don't get him here." The judge added that he expected "deference to this court," drawing a smile from some of the defense attorneys. "Don't smile, this is a serious matter," Hoffman said, before scolding one defense lawyer for turning his back to the judge. After the hearing, Ivy wrote to Miles Robinson that he was "quite positive that we can never obtain a fair trial with Judge Hoffman," adding that the judge had "acted like an insane person."[32]

The trial finally began with jury selection in late April as tensions brewed among the defendants and their lawyers (the defendants were represented by different attorneys). Ivy's lawyer, John Sembower, failed to get Ivy tried separately from the Durovics; Sembower had said that the jury might not be able to distinguish whatever evidence existed against Ivy from the "huge segments of evidence" that might be admitted against the brothers. Three of the attorneys who had been representing the Durovics withdrew from the case, charging that the brothers had not paid thousands of dollars in legal fees and had also made wild charges against the lawyers. "We were accused of working for the federal Food and Drug Administration," one attorney said. He added that he had "never lived through such an experience" and compared it to "a bad dream." Nonetheless, the jury was sworn in on April 30. The *Chicago Tribune* published the jurors' names and addresses and noted Judge Hoffman's repeated admonitions to the jurors not to follow any news coverage of the trial and not to discuss the case among themselves or with anyone else.[33]

Opening arguments took place a few days later. Assistant US attorney Thomas James told the jury that Krebiozen was "put to extensive commercial use for profit" at a time when the drug was supposed to be distributed only for experimental purposes. James said that Krebiozen's sponsors had deliberately and massively overstated the true costs of manufacturing the medicine. They also had lied when they said that Krebiozen was made from horse plasma; in reality, Krebiozen was creatine, and creatine could not be derived from plasma. Defense attorney Julius Sherwin countered that the government's charges of a conspiracy to defraud Krebiozen patients were grossly misdirected. "The real conspiracy in this case," said Sherwin, "is among small people in the Health, Education, and Welfare department and persons in a nationally recognized medical organization," that unnamed organization clearly being the AMA. Sherwin added that these "small people" had sought "to prevent, to defame, and to scuttle what may be the discovery of the century."[34]

Before the trial began, a US attorney had said that the government planned to call twenty witnesses; in fact, it would put more than one hundred people on the stand. As the prosecution slowly built its case, the defense repeatedly moved for a mistrial, making twenty-five such motions in the first six weeks of the proceedings. Judge Hoffman rejected them all. Notwithstanding Hoffman's cantankerousness, reporter William Woo commented that the judge "lent the one elegant tone to the trial" through his immaculate dress and precise delivery, with Hoffman "pronouncing words with the care a lapidary lavishes on precious stones." By way of contrast, Woo characterized prosecutor D. Arthur Connelly as a "short, edgy man" with white socks that "flashed like little flags" as he paced the courtroom. Ivy seemed to dress down for the trial by wearing a loose-fitting brown suit and cowboy boots. He regularly turned his chair toward the jury and away from his codefendants, including Stevan Durovic, who carried a cane that he periodically tapped and twirled during the proceedings. Stevan and his brother Marko each fell ill at different points during the trial—Marko with strep throat and Stevan with a kidney infection—which forced courtroom recesses. Judge Hoffman ordered a medical examination of Marko when defense attorney Sherwin claimed that he was near death. After a doctor reported that Marko's condition was not nearly so dire, the judge ordered him to return to the courtroom.[35]

One of the government's star witnesses was FDA investigator Robert Palmer, who was on the stand for more than two weeks. "I have never seen the government get such a runaround in all of my experience," he said of his months-long tussle with Ivy and the Durovics. Palmer said that Stevan had told him "that because of past experience they had learned how to be fighters, and if the government wanted to fight, the government would live to regret it." Other prosecution witnesses included NCI director Kenneth Endicott, FDA chemist Alma LeVant Hayden, and FDA reviewer Frances Oldham Kelsey, who had won fame for preventing thalidomide from reaching the US market. Defense attorney Sherwin objected to Kelsey's testimony, saying that the government was trying to portray Krebiozen as a "fellow traveler" of thalidomide.[36]

The prosecution rested its case in early October, whereupon the defense moved for immediate acquittal of all the defendants. After Judge Hoffman denied the motion, the defense proceeded to call fifty-seven witnesses of its own. Dr. John Pick spoke of Krebiozen's therapeutic powers, as did Gary Cathcart, who had started taking the drug as a boy in Wyoming and then had grown up to become a Rhodes scholar. Scott Anderson, a member of Senator Douglas's independent research group, testified for three days. He charged that the FDA had deliberately manipulated its spectrograms to make it seem as though Krebiozen and creatine were identical, whereas Krebiozen actually contained between 17 and 24 percent of some other substance. Anderson's testimony was often dense. He later recalled that he "went into a good lecture on physics, discussing the Beer-Lambert Law for the attenuation of a light beam passing through an absorbing medium." Before the trial, Ivy had unsuccessfully tried to prevent a jury consisting of laypersons from hearing the Krebiozen case on the grounds that such a jury would not be scientifically competent to evaluate the drug's merits. Although it was highly unlikely that the jurors who ended up hearing the case grasped all the nuances of what Anderson had said, he did help plant reasonable doubt in their minds about the prosecution's case against the defendants.[37]

The defense played on fears of government overreach, particularly with respect to the FDA. Prior to the trial, a California woman whose son had used Krebiozen wrote to Ivy that FDA investigators had visited her multiple times to tell her that she would be "aiding and abetting in a criminal act" by receiving the drug. "I'm sure you know that all I can think of is that by trying to keep our boy alive they have made me feel like a criminal," the woman told Ivy. The defense also charged the FDA with entrapment for having sent fake letters to the Krebiozen Research Foundation to try to document violations of federal drug laws. After a courtroom speech by one defense attorney railing against the government's methods, a pro-Krebiozen spectator burst into applause, and Judge Hoffman held him in contempt of court until he apologized. Outside the courtroom, Krebiozen supporters hurled abuse at FDA investigator Palmer, with one person telling him, "I hope you die a horrible death from cancer."[38]

The Durovic brothers and William Phillips never were called to testify, but Ivy took the stand as the star defense witness at the beginning of December. When the court clerk asked him to swear to tell the truth, the whole truth, and nothing but the truth, he replied, "Yes, provided I'm given the opportunity to tell the whole truth." Judge Hoffman asked the clerk to administer the oath again, to which Ivy merely said, "I do." He proceeded to recite a list of his many scientific accomplishments and accolades, prompted by his attorney John Sembower (he reportedly had told Sembower exactly what to ask him on the stand). Ivy even wheeled a cart filled with his awards into the courtroom. As his testimony continued over the next several days, Ivy told of how the White House had authorized a committee to evaluate Krebiozen, neglecting to mention how he and Stevan Durovic had sabotaged that committee. He showed test tubes of what he said were creatine and Krebiozen, and he noted that they were different colors. He also said that Kenneth Endicott had broken a promise that the NCI would conduct a fair test of the drug. Whatever his initial misgivings about the trial, Ivy had become confident and relaxed enough to curl up on a courtroom bench during a recess and take a nap, using his briefcase as a pillow.[39]

Then the prosecution's cross-examination began. Ivy acknowledged that he had never been on a hospital staff, had never removed a cancer, and had not performed a human operation of any kind since 1922. He admitted that the size of one woman's malignant tumor had increased by 80 to 90 percent after she began taking Krebiozen, but he denied that he had exaggerated the drug's efficacy by falsely reporting that Krebiozen patients had died for reasons other than cancer. When US attorney Connelly asked Ivy about a large sum of cash that had been deposited in his bank account, Ivy replied that he had earned it honestly through the stock market. Sembower and fellow defense attorney Sherwin each immediately moved for a mistrial because of what Sherwin called the "nasty unsupported inference" that Ivy had made the money from Krebiozen. Once more, Judge Hoffman rejected the defense motions, and the defense rested its case just before Christmas. The trial already had lasted longer than any previous criminal proceeding in Chicago federal district court.[40]

Closing arguments began in January 1966. Representing the prosecution, Connelly read aloud to the jury Hans Christian Andersen's "The Emperor's New Clothes": the tale of a vainglorious emperor fooled by two swindlers who pretend to weave for the emperor a magic set of clothes that supposedly are visible only to those individuals wise and worthy enough to see them. The swindlers abscond with bags full of silk and golden thread, while the emperor is left stripped and humiliated for all the world to see, although he never acknowledges his own foolishness. Connelly told the jury that Krebiozen was just such a fairy tale. He poured four ounces of ether into a bottle, producing fumes that made one juror cough repeatedly. Connelly noted that the defendants claimed to have poured "twelve hundred times that much ether down a drain" with "no odors, no dangers. That stuff is more explosive than gasoline, and yet they want you and me to believe that this is the process that they used to manufacture Krebiozen—the stuff in the fairy tale that just doesn't exist." The prosecutor said that most Krebiozen shipped over the years had contained only mineral oil. While being investigated by the FDA in 1963, the defendants had added creatine to the oil; as Connelly put it, "they had to come up with something." As for Ivy—the "emperor" in the Krebiozen tale—Connelly argued that perhaps he "could not conceive that he was wrong and would rather sell the American public down the river, so to speak, in order to protect his own ego and his pride." The prosecutor added that Ivy also might have been motivated by simple greed.[41]

Sharp differences had arisen among the defense attorneys during the trial, especially over whether William Phillips could be called to testify on Ivy's behalf, which Phillips's attorney had successfully opposed. Now, though, the attorneys were united in calling for acquittal of their clients. Julius Sherwin, who represented Marko Durovic, said that the defendants were on trial "for wanting to alleviate the scourge of cancer," and he predicted that one day they would "be compared to the martyrs of medicine." Edward Calihan, lawyer for Stevan Durovic, charged that the AMA had "never intended for Krebiozen to be scientifically evaluated" and had sought "to destroy Krebiozen." He added that "a finding of guilty on any one count will forever throw Krebiozen into oblivion." Ivy's attorney John Sembower read to the jury a different children's tale—Lewis Carroll's "The Walrus and the Carpenter"—and he implied that the agencies of organized medicine were much like the unscrupulous walrus and carpenter who had devoured the innocent oysters in Carroll's poem. The defendants had trusted those medical agencies to give Krebiozen a fair test, only to be betrayed. "Think of all the persons who suffered and died needlessly if Krebiozen is the answer!" Sembower said. Phillips's attorney Maurice Walsh asked the jury for a not guilty verdict on behalf of "the sick, the pain-racked, the desperate and dying. They will bless your name. . . . Your verdict will be a milestone in medicine and law, and it will be a message of hope to all those who have helped their fellow men."[42]

Judge Hoffman gave his charge to the jury. "This case bristles with issues of veracity," he said. "It is your function to decide where the truth lies." The jurors retired for what would become several days of deliberations, spending their waking hours in the jury room and their sleeping hours at the Palmer House hotel, where they were sequestered until they reached their verdicts. Krebiozen partisans—some of them wearing buttons saying, "I Need Krebiozen to Live!"—waited expectantly. Over the trial's duration, they had made their case for the drug to anyone who would listen. "My daughter has been taking Krebiozen for six years," one woman told a reporter. "She has a husband now and is going to have a baby. Without Krebiozen, she'd be dead. Ask her if it doesn't do any good!" The woman's daughter, who was standing wanly nearby, demurred: "Mother, I don't think I can go through this again."[43]

After deliberating for more than forty hours, the jury announced on January 29 that it had reached decisions on some, but not all, of the defendants. The courtroom was quickly packed with spectators, and the atmosphere was tense. Judge Hoffman cautioned everyone present to refrain from any demonstrations. Finally, the court clerk read aloud the verdicts: "We the jury find the defendant Andrew C. Ivy not guilty on all counts of the indictment." The clerk read similar not guilty verdicts for Marko Durovic and William Phillips. There were as of yet no verdicts for either Stevan Durovic or the Krebiozen Research Foundation, and the jury retired once more to resume its deliberations. A celebration immediately erupted outside the courtroom. "I feel very good. I always had hoped that things would turn out right," Ivy told reporters, as Krebiozen supporters swarmed around him.

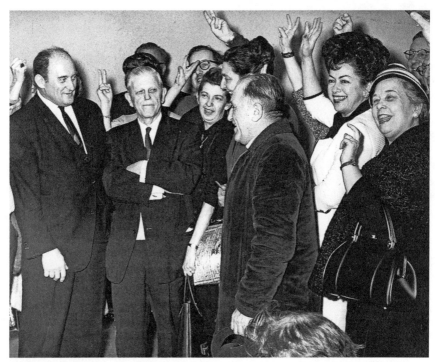

Andrew Ivy (second from left) surrounded by jubilant Krebiozen supporters after Ivy's acquittal in his fraud trial in January 1966. (Chicago Tribune/TCA)

Stevan Durovic, who at first appeared angry that the jury had not acquitted him along with everyone else, later managed a smile and said that he was happy with the verdicts so far.[44]

In the meantime, Durovic continued to wait. The jury deliberations came to an abrupt halt when one juror was hauled away on a stretcher, stricken with what was later said to be a combination of asthma and hypertension. She rejoined her fellow jurors after receiving treatment, and, on January 31, the jury announced its final verdicts: not guilty for both Durovic and the Krebiozen Research Foundation. Once more, Krebiozen proponents were jubilant, and some sobbed with joy. Gertrude Brou, the Florida woman had moved to Chicago so that she could continue to receive the drug, hugged Durovic. Jury foreman Adolph Beranek told reporters that some jurors had felt that Durovic "should not get away completely since he got money in promotion of the drug." However, they ultimately decided that if they did find him guilty, "it would kill Krebiozen. Most of us felt Krebiozen has a value and didn't want to hurt it." Beranek added that he believed that the government never should have prosecuted the case and that the money spent on the trial "could have been put to a better use, such as a laboratory test of the drug."[45]

Judge Hoffman was infuriated by the jury's verdicts. He also had been infuriated by the defense's tactics, particularly those of Julius Sherwin, who had told Hoffman that he was acting more like a prosecutor than a judge; Hoffman had gone as far as to draw up contempt papers against the lawyer. Concerning the jury, however, the judge had good reason to believe that there had been tampering. During the trial, jurors had received mailings from Krebiozen proponents, including from Kitty Schumacher of Scranton, Pennsylvania. Schumacher also had written pro-Krebiozen letters to Hoffman himself. She said that she had subscribed to the Chicago newspapers to follow the trial, and it was through those papers that she had found the jurors' home addresses. In her mailings, Schumacher included a copy of a letter from Patrick Gorman, who was head of the Amalgamated Meat Cutters and Butcher Workmen of North America and a revered figure in the labor movement. Gorman had taken up Krebiozen's cause, with his union's Chicago headquarters even displaying a pro-Krebiozen billboard. He had written to Schumacher about Krebiozen's support among organized labor and had railed against the "czardom" of the AMA. Schumacher had forwarded this letter to the jurors without Gorman's knowledge. She later said that the prosecution's likening of Krebiozen to a fairy tale "so infuriated me that I immediately decided I would send the letters to the jury."[46]

Although the jurors said that they had reported the letters to Judge Hoffman, they did not report that some of them also had discussed Krebiozen's merits throughout the trial, in direct violation of the judge's orders. *St. Louis Post-Dispatch* reporter Robert Collins discovered that a jury faction had continually belittled government witnesses and attorneys and made such comments as "the FDA is out to get everybody." Adolph Beranek had lobbied for the drug long before deliberations began. As one juror put it, "Mr. Beranek said he had read everything he could get on Krebiozen in case his wife, who had cancer, ever needed it, and he indicated he was very much in favor of the drug." Another juror, Joseph Bukowski, was on the Amalgamated Meat Cutters' executive board. He had attended a union convention in Springfield, Illinois, where Laine Friedman had delivered a speech extolling Krebiozen. Bukowski also had shown an issue of his union's magazine to his fellow jurors; the magazine had contained pro-Krebiozen articles. During deliberations, Bukowski became the fiercest proponent for acquittal. "His manner was rough, and he used strong language," a fellow juror remembered. Bukowski himself recalled that five jurors held out for convictions: "We had to work on the five and vice versa, but you know who won." According to US marshal Eugene Bissell, two male jurors had asked whether he could get them whiskey and prostitutes while the jury was sequestered at the Palmer House. Bissell believed that the jurors were deliberately trying to taint the government's case against the defendants: they could have reported that the government was trying to bribe them with sex and alcohol.[47]

Bukowski eventually stood trial for criminal contempt of court before Judge Hoffman. After a jury found Bukowski guilty, his wife screamed "you little Caesar!" at the judge, and other family members had to restrain her from lunging toward the bench. Hoffman sentenced Bukowski to three years in prison, saying that he had "flouted the dignity and authority of the federal court and the federal jury system," and he had been "convicted not only beyond a reasonable doubt, but beyond any doubt whatsoever." Kitty Schumacher was tried on similar charges before a different judge. She successfully argued that she had not known that she was doing anything wrong, and she was acquitted.[48]

While the jury shenanigans were coming to light, the government was filing new charges against Stevan Durovic, this time for filing false tax returns that had underreported his income by more than a million dollars. Durovic had no intention of answering the charges in person. Federal officials had seized his passport when he was first indicted in late 1964, but they returned it to him in early 1966 after the not guilty verdicts in the fraud trial. That move proved to be a mistake. Although federal agents were stationed at multiple airports to try to stop Durovic, he managed to evade them, flying first to Miami, then to the Bahamas, then to Bermuda, then to London, and finally to Paris. His brother Marko, who had stayed behind in Illinois, insisted that Stevan had left the country to seek emergency medical treatment: "He is a very sick man. He is very bad. His temperature keeps going up and down. He has a bad heart. Yes, I am sure he will return here to face the income tax charges if he recovers." It soon became apparent that Stevan's European sojourn would continue indefinitely. Meanwhile, he and Marko faced accusations from Julius Sherwin that they had failed to pay him more than $11,000 in legal fees.[49]

One protracted legal dispute related to Krebiozen came to a quiet end. Ivy dropped his libel suit against George Stoddard in June 1966 after Stoddard acknowledged that it was "not my purpose to question Dr. Ivy's integrity, sincerity, or dedication to scientific research." It had been eleven years since Ivy had first sued the former University of Illinois president for more than $300,000 in damages; in the end, he collected nothing.[50]

Krebiozen proponents mounted a last, determined effort to strike back at the drug's opponents and force the government to permit full access to the drug. Dr. Allen Rutherford and several cancer patients filed a lawsuit in federal district court against the AMA, the FDA, and both current and former U of I officials, including Stoddard. The plaintiffs claimed that the defendants had undertaken "a studied course of action and effective propaganda to destroy a medical remedy for cancer" in order to protect "the vast income presently received by the medical establishment" through its expensive, mainstream cancer treatments. The suit failed. After Senator Paul Douglas and ten fellow senators pressed the FDA to evaluate Krebiozen anew, the new FDA commissioner, James Goddard, told members of Congress that "mineral oil in itself may be carcinogenic." Goddard already had issued a statement declaring that despite the not guilty verdicts in the fraud

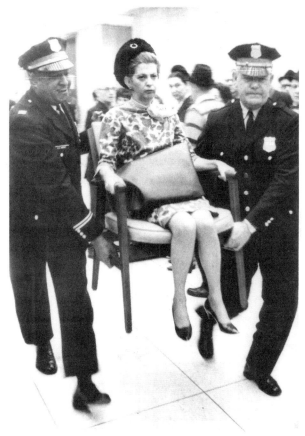

Gertrude Brou being carried away from a sit-in protest at the FDA's offices in March 1966. The protestors failed to get the FDA to reverse its stance on Krebiozen. (STM-036538891, Chicago Sun-Times Collection, Chicago History Museum)

trial, the FDA never would budge from its anti-Krebiozen stance: "There are 198 million people whose health and safety depend in some measure on the integrity of the FDA. For the sake of those 198 million people we *must* be forthright. We *must* adhere to the findings of science."[51]

A group of at least forty Krebiozen proponents staged one more sit-in in Washington, targeting Goddard's FDA office in March 1966. "Some of us won't be around next year," one of the protestors said, to which a fellow protestor replied, "A lot of us are dead already." Goddard refused to meet with the group, and, at the end of the business day, an FDA representative told the protestors that they had to leave. They refused. Laine Friedman, who was part of the group, called what happened next "one of the darkest hours of the Food and Drug Administration." Police yanked Max Rosenthal of Brooklyn, New York, from the corridor outside Goddard's office. They next moved toward Irvin Lieberman, who had virtually abandoned his business in Akron, Ohio, in order to devote his full energies to Krebiozen. Lieberman was carried into an elevator, down to the building lobby, and out to the street. Other protestors, some of them screaming and crying, began to leave on their own, but Gertrude Brou would not budge from her chair. She, too, was picked up and hauled away, chair and all.[52]

If it was a final, dramatic gesture on behalf of the drug, it also was a futile one. The acquittals in the fraud trial did the medicine no good. With Stevan Durovic now in Europe, Krebiozen became scarce, and it soon faded from the news. The drug stayed legal in Illinois for a few more years through a loophole that allowed drugs that had been manufactured in the state prior to 1969 to remain available. In the fall of 1973, a new state law closed that loophole and made Krebiozen illegal; soon thereafter, the US Supreme Court let stand a lower court ruling that blocked marketing of the drug. Twenty-two years after Andrew Ivy's announcement of a new and strikingly promising cancer medicine, Krebiozen was effectively dead.[53]

What Ever Happened to Doctor Ivy?

Andrew Ivy never gave up on Krebiozen; at least, he never gave up on the idea of a Krebiozen-like drug. In February 1967, a little more than a year after his acquittal in the fraud trial, Ivy was feted in Chicago at a dinner celebrating his seventy-fourth birthday. He was introduced at the dinner by his onetime pupil Dr. George Crane, who, after medical school, had gone on to write a nationally syndicated newspaper column promoting conservativism. (Crane's sons Phil and Dan would both enter Republican politics and represent Illinois in Congress.) Crane would use his column to help Ivy promote a new drug called Carcalon, which seemed to be essentially the same as the "lipopolysaccharide C" substance that Ivy previously had touted as a generic equivalent to Krebiozen. Ivy told the audience at his birthday dinner that he now was deliberately avoiding the "Krebiozen" label because the Food and Drug Administration still claimed jurisdiction over that drug, whereas, according to Ivy, Carcalon was free from FDA oversight. He added that he never would sell Carcalon, but instead would dispense it for free, with financial contributions from Ivy Cancer Leagues across the country helping to ensure its continued availability. In another similarity to Krebiozen, the name "Carcalon" was said to come from the ancient Greek words "karkos" and "chalone," connoting a natural cancer suppressor.[1]

A few months after the birthday dinner, Roosevelt University in Chicago informed Ivy that he would have to vacate his laboratory in the Auditorium Building tower. During the fraud trial, Roosevelt officials had been sensitive to the potential embarrassment that Ivy might bring to the university, but they had chosen to do nothing that might call additional attention to the situation, adhering to what one official called "the old administrative principle of 'prudent neglect'." Now, though, the university said that it needed to renovate Ivy's lab space to accommodate other needs, and it did not seem eager to renew the five-year agreement that it had made with him back in 1962 designating him as an unsalaried research professor. Ivy moved his lab to a new space in the Chicago Loop, with the costs once more underwritten by donations from the Ivy Cancer Leagues. He said that he was administering Carcalon (derived from horse serum, again like Krebiozen) to about eighty cancer patients each month, all from Illinois; despite his bravado about the FDA not controlling his work, the FDA had said that the interstate distribution ban on Krebiozen also applied to Carcalon.[2]

Ivy may have avoided conviction in federal court, but his scientific reputation was in tatters, just as it had been almost from the time that he first embraced Krebiozen. An oft-repeated story maintained that, shortly before Anton Carlson died in 1956, he spoke sadly about Ivy, his onetime protégé. "Thank God my trouble is here," said Carlson while pointing to his heart, "instead of *here*"—and Carlson pointed to his head, implying that Ivy had gone crazy. In 1959, the American Physiological Society met at the University of Illinois while Ivy still worked there; Ivy once had served as the society's president. A fellow physiologist remembered conversing with Ivy at the entrance to a large venue where a barbecue was about to take place: "As usual, Ivy talked at length about Krebiozen. We stood in the wide doorway, he with his back to those entering. I noticed several coming in who I knew had been Ivy's friends and admirers. None stopped to speak with us; it seemed to me they were intent on avoiding Ivy." For his part, Ivy denied having lost any real friends over Krebiozen, saying that "it is only the people who have been brainwashed who may not be my friends." Yet the *New York Post* said that he seemed to have become "a very lonely man," and *Life* magazine—in its story "What Ever Happened to Dr. Ivy?"—suggested that the fallout over Krebiozen had ruined him: "His great laboratory days are now long behind him, his high posts and fabulous prestige in his profession are dim in memory."[3]

• • •

What *did* happen to Andrew Ivy? For that matter, what happened to everyone else to keep the Krebiozen controversy raging for the better part of two decades?

There was no shortage of theories about Ivy. One such theory was that he had suffered a stroke or some other trauma or condition that had clouded his judgment and dimmed his mental faculties. In reality, Ivy showed no signs of dementia or other impairment. When asked about the idea that he had succumbed to madness, Ivy laughed. "I mentioned that rumor to Mrs. Ivy one time," he said, "and she said if I was off my rocker I've been off my rocker ever since she has known me, and that goes back forty-seven years." Another theory, which had been advanced by the prosecution during the fraud trial, was that Ivy had been motivated by avarice. However, *Life*'s story about him noted that he never had seemed to care much about money, and Ivy himself railed against the government's insinuations that his routine bank and stock transactions had somehow added up to his making a small fortune from Krebiozen. In any event, the government never claimed that Ivy had made anything close to the millions of dollars that Stevan Durovic was said to have acquired by soliciting almost ten dollars per ampule of the drug.[4]

According to *Life*, some of Ivy's erstwhile admirers believed that he had been duped by a master con artist. The "master" part of that assumption strained credulity. If Durovic believed that he had concocted a diabolical surefire scheme to defraud victims of medical maladies around the world, the scheme failed miserably the first time that he tried to spring it on physicians in the United States. A Northwestern University doctor had found Durovic to be laughably inept in his insistence that Kositerin cured hypertension, calling him "stupid beyond my ken." In the years that followed, most other medical professionals came to similar conclusions about Durovic and the cancer medicine that he called Krebiozen.[5]

Although it is still possible that Krebiozen was designed as an elaborate con from the start, it is also possible that Durovic, through a mixture of hubris and foolishness, convinced himself that he really had come up with a wonder drug that cured multiple ills: a close relative of Aleksandr Bogomolets's "ACS" medicine that, like Krebiozen, was derived from horse blood and was credited during the 1940s as being effective against everything from arthritis to cancer. In Argentina, Durovic's drug attracted the support of Juan Perón's regime, which had a proclivity for self-promotion through new inventions and medicines.[6] The regime's backing of Durovic's medicine drew the attention of two US businesspeople, R. Edwin Moore and Kenneth Brainard, who then brought Durovic to Chicago. The goal seemed to be winning the support of a major university medical center: a novel strategy for promoters of an unproven remedy. Whereas the likes of John Brinkley and Norman Baker had turned to radio to boost their nostrums, Durovic and his American sponsors sought the scholarly and scientific prestige associated with the postwar research university. That strategy relied on persuading a high-profile scientist to endorse the nostrum. Northwestern University's doctors did not take the bait; Andrew Ivy did.

After Durovic managed to ensnare Ivy, Stevan's brother Marko also came to Chicago, determined to protect the family's financial interests against outsiders just as he had done with the brothers' business partners in Argentina. If money was to be made from Stevan's drug, whether it be named Kositerin or Krebiozen, the Durovics were determined that it would be made by them. The battle over money led to much of the turmoil that followed over Krebiozen. As U of I president George Stoddard put it at the time, there appeared to be "a scramble to get on the financial band wagon and then perhaps a falling out over dividing the profits expected to follow upon a dramatic presentation by a renowned scientist of 'an agent for the treatment of malignant tumors'."[7]

But how was Stevan able to ensnare Ivy to begin with and prompt him to make his 1951 announcement of Krebiozen at the Drake Hotel? Rather than being infirm, greedy, or improbably naïve, Ivy seemed to be driven more by ambition and his legendary stubbornness. One doctor would comment that, by the late 1940s, Ivy had become "dissatisfied with the degree of his contribution to science." Having a strong appetite for publicity, he "regularly made statements to the newspapers on numerous subjects, and though he thus became very popular and very successful as a money-raiser, his scientific colleagues had already become a shade suspicious." For example, they were skeptical of Ivy's claims for a device called a "flicker photometer" that he had devised with his colleague Louis Krasno; the device supposedly revealed early signs of heart disease by detecting a narrowing in the retinal arteries. When Durovic showed up at Ivy's office with claims for a medicine that harnessed the body's natural defenses against cancer, Ivy was intrigued, for it aligned with his own theories about that medical condition—and, not incidentally, there could be no greater contribution to science than an effective, noninvasive, and nontoxic treatment for cancer. Thus, Ivy directed Krasno to try Durovic's drug on human subjects. When the results seemed promising, Ivy's commitment to Krebiozen was secured.[8]

That his commitment remained unshaken, despite all the personal and professional travails that he suffered, was testament of Ivy's willfulness, if not arrogance. "There are different types of stubbornness," he once told an interviewer. "One type is 'obstinate prejudice' where the individual will not change his mind, no matter what the facts are. He's like the sign that says, 'My mind is made up. Don't confuse me with the facts.'" In contrast, Ivy insisted that he displayed tenacity, a stubborn devotion to the facts that had been characteristic of Louis Pasteur and all the other legendary scientists. Ivy had concluded that the evidence showed that Krebiozen was scientifically valuable and deserved a fair test, notwithstanding that he was not a specialist well versed in cancer's unpredictable course or the variable responses of patients to purported treatments. "I have never made a conclusion shown to be wrong," Ivy told the interviewer. "You have to read my conclusions carefully because the words are carefully selected. I do not go beyond the facts." Pursuing the facts as he saw them was his "scientific duty."[9] So Ivy dug in for the long haul, refusing to be budged by the negative pronouncements of organized medicine that came from the American Medical Association, the National Research Council, the Chicago Medical Society, the U of I's Cole Committee, the American Cancer Society, the Food and Drug Administration, and the National Cancer Institute. The Durovics, of course, were not about to try to dissuade Ivy from his support of Krebiozen, and when Stevan struggled to keep up with the growing demand for the drug, he was not about to admit that in most cases there was nothing in the ampules but mineral oil.

Without Ivy's prestige and political connections, the Krebiozen controversy would have quickly fizzled. The drug emerged from a unique set of historical conditions, with a flagship public state university seeking to revitalize itself and achieve preeminence in the immediate postwar era. Those conditions are what brought Ivy to the U of I to begin with; he was one of many attention-grabbing hires of star professors that the university splurged on during those years. But the pace of change sparked by the new generation of administrators, faculty, and students deeply unsettled many people. The first years of the Cold War—as Russia detonated an atomic bomb, communists took power in China, war erupted in Korea, and Joseph McCarthy launched his red-baiting campaign—compounded anxieties. The rise of the postwar "multiversity" meant that major universities such as the U of I increasingly would have to answer to multiple publics and competing interests, with university presidents expected to play the role of mediator.[10] George Stoddard at that point of his academic career did not seem inclined to try to smooth over all the tensions that arose during his administration. As the most visible symbol of change at the U of I, he became a target of vilification, especially after internal squabbling in academic units attracted widespread publicity and heightened the questioning of his leadership. Krebiozen came along at precisely the right moment to be wielded against Stoddard and all that he represented. The drug's close association with Ivy, who had long cultivated the press and Illinois lawmakers, enhanced Krebiozen's potency as a political weapon, even if it was impotent against cancer.

After Stoddard was ousted, the Illinois legislature's Krebiozen committee no longer had the funds or motivation to continue its investigation indefinitely, and it disbanded. Yet the Krebiozen controversy persisted, in large part because the federal government did not immediately intervene.

The medicine appeared to fall in a gap between the authority of the FDA and the authority of the Public Health Service, taking advantage of the fact that nobody knew whether Krebiozen was a hormone or a serum or something else entirely. An AMA attorney who reviewed the regulatory history of the medicine opined that "Krebiozen's strong political sponsorship is the most likely reason why Krebiozen was not proceeded against" sooner by the government's medical agencies.[11]

The foremost political sponsor of the drug was US senator Paul Douglas of Illinois, who was markedly different from most of the other politicians who to that point had championed Krebiozen. As a liberal Democrat, Douglas took positions much closer to those of Stoddard than to those of conservative state legislators who had fought to rid the university of Stoddard, and although Douglas's political roots were in Chicago, he had battled against the city's Democratic machine at least as often as he had defended its interests. His support of Krebiozen stemmed from his long friendship with Ivy and his profound distrust of what he viewed as the entrenched power of the AMA and FDA. In 1963, after the FDA exerted its new regulatory authority under the Kefauver-Harris Amendment by investigating Krebiozen and reporting it to be creatine, Douglas bitterly dismissed the FDA report, and he tried to circumvent it through the intercession of President Johnson. Even after Durovic and Ivy betrayed the senator's efforts, Douglas still refused to repudiate them or Krebiozen publicly.

The government, bolstered by the FDA's and NCI's scathing assessments of the medicine, proceeded to prosecute Ivy, Durovic, and other Krebiozen sponsors. The failure to secure a single guilty verdict likely stemmed in part from the government having made its case too complex and having framed its charges too broadly; it might have been more successful had it focused strictly on violations of federal drug laws without also trying to prove fraud.[12] Also working against the government, of course, was the jury's blatant disregard of the judge's instructions not to discuss the case, in addition to other jury tampering coming from outside the courtroom. But cultural factors played an important role, too: in particular, a populist view of medicine, or what James Harvey Young called a "view from below." Before Krebiozen came along, plenty of other quack cancer remedies had attracted widespread popular support, such as those peddled by Harry Hoxsey and William Frederick Koch. "No doubt, ignorance and desperation made some people easy prey for quack promotions," one historian writes. He adds, though, that for other people, such remedies were a reasoned choice: "After consulting others, comparing costs, and measuring religious convictions and common sense, many people came to view quack healers as a viable medical option."[13]

The same was true of Krebiozen, as populist mistrust of organized medicine merged with populist mistrust of other persons and institutions viewed as elitist or remote. The FDA's use of subterfuge in its Krebiozen investigation stirred ire, as did its badgering of certain cancer patients and their family members. Labor unions had reason to dislike the AMA, in that it had sought to undermine some unions' health insurance programs.[14] Unions defied the AMA's dismissal of Krebiozen by backing the drug, and labor's influence (improperly wielded by a juror and a pro-Krebiozen letter writer) reached into the jury room during the fraud trial.

In Illinois, many people had detested U of I president Stoddard not just for having imported faculty who taught such things as Keynesian economic theory instead of practical business training; they also had viewed Stoddard as an arrogant, autocratic outsider. State lawmakers such as Roland Libonati and Vito Marzullo—devotees of Chicago's peculiar brand of patronage politics—similarly disliked professors whom they viewed as overeducated eastern elites. "The university is not a place for carpetbaggers," Libonati said, while adding that he preferred people "who are not too expert."[15] To such individuals, support of Krebiozen came naturally. Journalists who prided themselves on their affinity to common folk were sympathetic to Krebiozen as well. Even if the journalists were skeptical of some of the claims made for the drug, Ivy's rapport with the press and his self-representation as a hardy midwestern man of the people encouraged them to support the kind of "fair test" that Ivy advocated.

Ivy appealed to more than just populist interests, however. His academic credentials worked in his favor by giving Krebiozen gravitas that earlier quack medicines could not match. It was far easier to view him as a modern-day Pasteur than it was viewing such hucksters as John Brinkley and Norman Baker as serious scientists. So it was that Herbert Bailey latched onto Ivy as an exemplar of a fearless scholar searching for the truth in the face of appalling greed and abuse of power. Proponents of nonmainstream therapies, such as Gloria Swanson, also found it easy to endorse Ivy's efforts on behalf of Krebiozen.

In particular, many people with cancer and their loved ones saw Krebiozen as a legitimate alternative—perhaps the only alternative. "I begged the doctors to give my husband radiation, anything," said Laine Friedman about her husband George. "But they rejected my pleas stating there was nothing that could help. It was then that I turned to Krebiozen." A woman whose mother had taken the drug for her cancer commented that it seemed to have given her "a few painless weeks, which is a great deal more than the medical profession did with surgery and X rays." No one was more dedicated to science than Rachel Carson, but, by her own account, her negative experiences with mainstream medicine had left her with "great cynicism about doctors." She researched Krebiozen enough to know that it would not cure her cancer, but she tried the drug anyway, hoping that she "might live more comfortably and perhaps somewhat longer than otherwise." Although Carson ultimately found no benefit from the medicine, other individuals who firmly believed that it was helping them seemed to experience a placebo effect from Krebiozen, even if in actuality it did nothing to stop the progression of their diseases. In such ways, the drug filled the role of what Harry Collins and Trevor Pinch have called medicine as succor.[16]

Krebiozen followed in multiple ways the pattern of quack medicines that had come before it and also set a template for quack medicines that came after it. The conspiracy charges that Krebiozen partisans directed at the AMA and other agencies of organized medicine had likewise been leveled by Brinkley, Baker, and Hoxsey in the past. The use of academic and scientific credentials to bolster the credibility of a quack drug was already familiar from Koch and his Glyoxylide medicine. The FDA's efforts in court to win a guilty verdict against Koch had failed, just as they also would fail with Ivy, Durovic, and Krebiozen.[17]

After Krebiozen finally fell into disfavor, amygdalin—better known as Laetrile—became the best-known nonmainstream cancer treatment. The controversy surrounding the drug in the 1970s was eerily reminiscent of the one that had surrounded Krebiozen. Once again, as the *New York Times* reported, pillars of government and organized medicine declared that Laetrile "was useless and the people behind it were classic cancer quacks who were taking advantage of frightened cancer victims." In response, Laetrile proponents "spoke of the medical-drug-company-Government 'conspiracy' to hold back a 'valid' anticancer substance from the public," and they "condemned the Establishment for arrogantly denying cancer victims the right to freely choose their mode of treatment." Once again, state lawmakers seized on the controversy, but on a much vaster scale than what had happened with Krebiozen; twenty-seven states legalized Laetrile even while the FDA banned its interstate shipment. Once again, a liberal Democratic US senator called for a fair scientific test of the drug, that senator being Edward Kennedy of Massachusetts. This time, the political pressure was such that the NCI and the FDA eventually approved a clinical trial of Laetrile. "No substantive benefit was observed in terms of cure, improvement, or stabilization of cancer, improvements of symptoms related to cancer, or extension of life span," the *New England Journal of Medicine* reported in 1982 of the trial's results. Moreover, the drug could lead to cyanide poisoning.[18]

In Laetrile's wake, a scientist even more renowned than Ivy became entangled in an unproven cancer remedy, as Nobel laureate Linus Pauling extolled the benefits of vitamin C. Other Nobel laureates have embraced out-of-the-mainstream ideas about race (as with William Shockley and James Watson), climate change, and autism, indicating that Ivy was hardly unique as a once-distinguished researcher who strayed from the tenets of evidence-based science. As one study has put it, "remarkable levels of intelligence" do not necessarily "immunize individuals against equally remarkable lapses in critical thinking."[19] Meanwhile, miracle diets and shark cartilage have been trumpeted as cancer therapies, and a Polish scientist named Stanislaw Burzynski has pushed "antineoplastons," a supposedly revolutionary treatment derived from human urine. None of those remedies has been proved to be effective against cancer.[20] The enduring appeal of such treatments seems to stem at least as much from hope as it does from fear. "When people in distress have a tremendous need to believe in something or somebody, then the forces of society seem powerless to effect an unmasking of the inconsistencies involved in that faith," physician John T. Flynn wrote in 1966 about Krebiozen. He added that "such vigor of faith no doubt is a necessity to many people in their times of crisis."

The danger, said Flynn, comes when "constant repetition of unsubstantiated statements eventually produces the appearance of truth."[21] That danger is as acute today as ever, with widespread misinformation and disinformation about COVID-19 and other medical conditions, renewed attacks on science and public education, and populist politics degenerating into demagoguery. The story of Krebiozen is a poignant reminder that those travails are nothing new, but instead have ample historical precedent. It is also a reminder of the damage that can be inflicted when quackery and all the untruths that accompany it go unchecked for too long.

• • •

George Stoddard resuscitated his academic career after being forced to leave the University of Illinois. He served in leadership roles at New York University and at Long Island University before retiring in 1969. Even after that, he still was trying to make sense of Krebiozen, and, in 1971, he wrote an outline for a play or novel inspired by the bizarre history of the drug. There was a "Dr. Dvago," who brings a mysterious emphysema medicine to the United States by way of South America; a "Senator Wavering," who gives the medicine his political backing; and a "Dr. X," who "thus far has never made a scientific or medical discovery that has held up. Nor has he, in his mind, ever made a mistake." Dr. X decides that Dvago's drug "is too good, too powerful, too wonderful for emphysema—only a cure for cancer is worthy for such a scientific find." It will bring him the fame and vindication that he believes he richly deserves. Dvago, in turn, "gleams like a cat that sees its helpless prey and is ready to seize it." The drug is eventually revealed to be nothing but rubbing alcohol with a pinch of baking soda. In the end, with Dvago now "rich and absent," Dr. X is reduced to treating children afflicted with chicken pox, while the people who had placed their hopes in Dvago's elixir resignedly "return to honest diagnosis and treatment." Stoddard never developed his outline further, and he died in 1981.[22]

In his public comments on the Krebiozen affair, Stoddard had been particularly bitter toward US senator Paul Douglas. Stoddard called Douglas's support of Krebiozen "reprehensible. He's a former university professor himself and should know what scientific protocol is." In 1966, a few months after the Krebiozen fraud trial ended, Douglas was defeated in his bid for a fourth Senate term by Illinois Republican Charles Percy. Douglas then wrote his memoirs, in which he expressed his disillusionment with the FDA and other federal agencies that he said had been guilty of "bureaucratic injustice." Not once, however, did he mention Andrew Ivy or Krebiozen. When Douglas died in 1976, the *Chicago Tribune*, which over the years had looked askance at his liberalism, saluted him for always having been "his own man. He put his foot down for what he thought was right, no matter whose toes got in the way."[23]

Marko Durovic, who, along with his brother Stevan, had gained permanent-resident status in the United States thanks largely to Douglas, successfully defended himself against federal tax-fraud charges in 1970. He was arrested the following year at his home in the Chicago suburb of Winnetka for having failed to pay more than three hundred parking tickets. The police officers who took him into custody reported that Marko "read us a long lecture, saying that he had a law degree in France and that we were forbidden to make an arrest without a warrant and after eight o'clock at night. We told him he wasn't in France." Marko ended up being fined a little more than $1,500. He died in 1976, not long after Douglas's death.[24]

Stevan Durovic, while facing his own tax charges, had stolen away to France in 1966 shortly after being acquitted in the Krebiozen trial. He soon left Paris for Switzerland, which, coincidentally or not, was where one of his overseas bank accounts was located. Marko told a reporter that Stevan was being treated for tuberculosis at a Swiss sanitarium. "If my brother doesn't die, he will come back to the United States," Marko said. Stevan survived, but he never returned to America. According to available records, he outlived the other principals in the Krebiozen affair by several years, dying in Geneva in 1988 just shy of his eighty-third birthday.[25]

Andrew Ivy continued to treat cancer patients with Carcalon until declining health forced him to retire a couple of years before his own death in 1978 at the age of eighty-four. Ivy gave one of his final interviews to Chicago newspaper columnist Jack Mabley, a longtime friend. "Ninety percent of my patients have been written off," Ivy told Mabley. "It's the blood of your heart to see some of the people come in. Most of them have had their cells, their whole defense mechanism, destroyed by toxic cancer suppressives. But if there's a chance of their being helped by traditional methods, I advise them to see a surgeon. I treat them only when they won't take anything else. What am I going to do—kick them out?" Mabley also talked to Catherine Manning, who had loyally served as executive director of the Ivy Cancer Research Foundation for many years. Her assessment of Ivy was heartfelt and succinct: "He keeps working, he does no harm, and he has faith."[26]

Ivy's devotion and faith in his work were beyond question. Wanting to further the cause of medicine by investigating ways in which the human body defends itself against cancer was, of course, a worthy and important endeavor; other scientists who later undertook such work would make significant research breakthroughs. It is clear that Ivy truly believed that he was helping people with Krebiozen, and that belief surely motivated him at least as much as his quest for scientific acclaim.

Yet it was a vast misstatement to suggest that Ivy had done no harm. He had abused his status as a respected academic and scientific expert in his vigorous endorsement of Krebiozen. His acceptance of sketchy, second-hand data on Krebiozen patients, his refusal to consider more scientifically plausible explanations of the drug's ostensible effects, his unwillingness to challenge Durovic's secrecy surrounding Krebiozen or the exorbitant prices being charged for the drug, and his complicity with the conspiracy charges brandished against Krebiozen's opponents all had a devastating impact. A history of the U of I's medical programs notes that "as the Krebiozen controversy dragged on, morale fell, faculty resigned, student applications decreased and progress in other areas was overshadowed."[27] The reputation of the entire university suffered as well. For a time, the not-guilty verdicts for Ivy and Durovic made the FDA leery of pursuing antifraud investigations; as one FDA representative recalled, "every time you would get hold of something involving quackery, the first thing everybody would scream would be, 'We don't want another Krebiozen on our hands.'"[28] Most important, some people with cancer who might have benefited from mainstream treatments chose to forgo them in favor of taking an unproven and ultimately discredited remedy.

However, Ivy might have achieved a small measure of redemption late in his life. When he gave his Krebiozen-like drug for free to people with terminal cancer, he also gave them a chance to feel that they were doing something proactive and meaningful at a time when standard treatments could no longer save them. In essence, Ivy was providing them with compassion that not only did them no real harm, but also likely did them some good. "There are three aspects of a physician's service to a patient," Ivy said at that time. "One is science or knowledge; a second is skill in the application of knowledge and experience; the other is sympathy and hope. The latter is sometimes all that we can offer the patient." As *Life* magazine put it, even after Ivy had been professionally disgraced, he still was dispensing "an old-fashioned brand of medical sympathy out of a forgotten age."[29]

Organized medicine's seeming lack of sympathy is one reason that people turn to unproven remedies, according to medical professor F. Perry Wilson in his 2023 book *How Medicine Works and When It Doesn't*. Wilson says that reforming health care to make it more affordable and accessible can enhance trust in mainstream medicine. But he also argues that the system needs to change to allow doctors to spend more time with patients and make them feel that they have been truly listened to and cared for. "It turns out that sometimes you need something to hang on to—a dash of hope, a soupçon of meaning—to keep you moving forward one day at a time," says Wilson. His words echo those of Dr. George Crile Jr. back in the 1950s when the Krebiozen controversy first erupted: "If physicians, in an age that is thought of as being an age of science, devote themselves solely to the scientific side of medical practice, if they fail to inspire their patients with hope and faith, it is not surprising that quackery flourishes."[30]

In pondering the story of Andrew Ivy and Krebiozen, then, we should remember what can happen when laudable faith in the power of medical discovery is tainted by misplaced ambition and obstinacy and coopted by individuals seeking financial and political profit. We should remember, too, that quackery will almost certainly always be with us, and we should be able to recognize its telltale signs whenever it occurs. But we also should never lose sight of the power of medicine as succor. Harnessing that power can be an important step toward reinforcing confidence in medicine as science. It might even reduce the likelihood of more Krebiozen-like sagas in the future.

Notes

Introduction

1. Philip H. Stoddard, "'The Giftie Gie Us,'" in George D. Stoddard, *The Pursuit of Education: An Autobiography* (New York: Vantage, 1981), 285.

2. "Citizen Doctor," *Time*, January 13, 1947, https://content.time.com/time/subscriber/article/0,33009,855589,00.html. See also Jerry Sohl, "Says New Cancer Drug May Be Greatest Medical Discovery," *Pantagraph* (Bloomington, IL), April 8, 1951, 3; A. C. Ivy, John F. Pick, and W. F. P. Phillips, *Observations on Krebiozen in the Management of Cancer* (Chicago: Henry Regnery, 1956), 5.

3. Sohl, "Says New Cancer Drug," 3.

4. George D. Stoddard, *"Krebiozen": The Great Cancer Mystery* (Boston: Beacon, 1955), 4.

5. Arthur L. Caplan, "Doctors, Scientists, Did the Quacks Get Your Tongue? Time to Take It Back," *Times Higher Education*, May 11, 2023, https://www.timeshighereducation.com/opinion/doctors-scientists-did-quacks-get-your-tongue-time-take-it-back.

6. Geoff Brumfiel, "Doubting Mainstream Medicine, COVID Patients Find Dangerous Advice and Pills Online," NPR.org, July 19, 2022, https://www.npr.org/sections/health-shots/2022/07/19/1111794832/doubting-mainstream-medicine-covid-patients-find-dangerous-advice-and-pills-onli. See also *Confronting Health Misinformation: The U.S. Surgeon General's Advisory on Building a Healthy Information Environment* (Washington, DC: United States Department of Health and Human Services, 2021), https://www.hhs.gov/sites/default/files/surgeon-general-misinformation-advisory.pdf.

7. Edward J. Balleisen, *Fraud: An American History from Barnum to Madoff* (Princeton, NJ: Princeton University Press, 2017), 5, 14; Gary E. Friedlaender and Linda K. Friedlaender, "Art in Science: Quackery and Promises Not Kept," *Clinical Orthopaedics and Related Research* 480, no. 8 (2022): 1458. See also Joe

Schwarcz, *Quack Quack: The Threat of Pseudoscience* (Toronto, ON: ECW Press, 2022).

8. Eric S. Juhnke, *Quacks and Crusaders: The Fabulous Careers of John Brinkley, Norman Baker, and Harry Hoxsey* (Lawrence: University Press of Kansas, 2002); R. Alton Lee, *The Bizarre Careers of John R. Brinkley* (Lexington: University Press of Kentucky, 2002); Pope Brock, *Charlatan: America's Most Dangerous Huckster, the Man Who Pursued Him, and the Age of Flimflam* (New York: Crown, 2008); John Carreyrou, *Bad Blood: Secrets and Lies in a Silicon Valley Startup* (New York: Alfred A. Knopf, 2018).

9. Juhnke, *Quacks and Crusaders*; James Harvey Young and Richard E. McFayden, "The Koch Cancer Treatment," *Journal of the History of Medicine and Allied Sciences* 53, no. 3 (July 1998): 254–84; James Harvey Young, *American Health Quackery: Collected Essays* (Princeton, NJ: Princeton University Press, 1992), 205–55; Evelleen Richards, *Vitamin C and Cancer: Medicine or Politics?* (Houndmills, UK: Macmillan, 1991); "List of Unproven and Disproven Cancer Treatments," Wikipedia.org, https://en.wikipedia.org/wiki/List_of_unproven _and_disproven_cancer_treatments. See also "Cancer Treatment Watch," *Quackwatch*, https://quackwatch.org/cancer/; Paul A. Offit, *Do You Believe in Magic? The Sense and Nonsense of Alternative Medicine* (New York: Harper, 2013), e-book, chaps. 2, 8–9.

10. Nina L. Shapiro, "Quackery and Hype: Mesmerized by Wizards," *Social Research* 85, no. 4 (Winter 2018): 889. See also Schwarcz, *Quack Quack*; Edzard Ernst, *So-Called Alternative Medicine (SCAM) for Cancer* (Cham, Switz.: Springer Nature, 2021); Balleisen, *Fraud*.

11. Young, *American Health Quackery*, 236–42 (emphasis added). See also William T. Jarvis and Stephen Barrett, "How Quackery Sells," in *The Health Robbers: A Close Look at Quackery in America,* edited by Stephen Barrett and William T. Jarvis, 1–22 (Buffalo, NY: Prometheus, 1993); "Understanding Cancer," National Cancer Institute, https://www.cancer.gov/about-cancer/understanding; "Cancer," *MedlinePlus*, last updated May 18, 2017, https://medlineplus.gov/ cancer.html; William G. Rothstein, *American Medical Schools and the Practice of Medicine: A History* (New York: Oxford University Press, 1987), 242.

12. Carreyrou, *Bad Blood*; David Streitfeld, "The Epic Rise and Fall of Elizabeth Holmes," *New York Times*, January 3, 2022, https://www.nytimes .com/2022/01/03/technology/elizabeth-holmes-theranos.html.

13. Matthew Hongoltz-Hetling, *If It Sounds like a Quack . . .: A Journey to the Fringes of American Medicine* (New York: Public Affairs, 2023), e-book, introduction, chap. 6; Schwarcz, *Quack Quack*, 231.

14. Morris Fishbein, "History of Cancer Quackery," *Perspectives in Biology and Medicine* 8, no. 2 (Winter 1965): 166; James T. Patterson, *The Dread Disease: Cancer and Modern American Culture* (Cambridge, MA: Harvard University Press, 1987); Siddhartha Mukherjee, *The Emperor of All Maladies: A Biography of Cancer* (New York: Scribner, 2011); Rebecca L. Siegel, Kimberly D. Miller, Nikita Sandeep Wagle, and Ahmedin Jemal, "Cancer Statistics, 2023," *CA*

73, no. 1 (January 2023): 17–48; Marlene Cimons, "Debunking Myths about Cancer," *Washington Post*, June 10, 2022, https://www.washingtonpost.com /health/2022/06/10/cancer-myths/; Libby Watson, "After the War on Cancer," *Baffler*, March 23, 2023, https://thebaffler.com/latest/after-the-war-on-cancer -watson; Kate Pickert, "Is a Revolution in Cancer Treatment within Reach?," *New York Times*, June 16, 2023, https://www.nytimes.com/2023/06/16/opinion /cancer-treatment-disparities.html; Azra Raza, *The First Cell: And the Human Costs of Pursuing Cancer to the Last* (New York: Basic Books, 2019), 6.

15. Susan Sontag, *Illness as Metaphor and AIDS and Its Metaphors* (New York: Picador, 2001), 58, 155. See also Philip Kennicott, "The Virus Caused More Than a Pandemic. It Set Us All Ablaze," *Washington Post*, February 5, 2021, https://www.washingtonpost.com/entertainment/coronavirus-pandemic-disease /2021/02/03/96a75d14–658a-11eb-8c64–9595888caa15_story.html.

16. F. Perry Wilson, *How Medicine Works and When It Doesn't: Learning Who to Trust to Get and Stay Healthy* (New York: Grand Central, 2023), e-book, chap. 7 (emphasis in original).

17. Stoddard, *Pursuit of Education*, 139.

18. Harry Collins and Trevor Pinch, *Dr. Golem: How to Think about Medicine* (Chicago: University of Chicago Press, 2005), e-book, introduction. See also Patterson, *Dread Disease*; John H. McArthur and Francis D. Moore, "The Two Cultures and the Health Care Revolution: Commerce and Professionalism in Medical Care," *Journal of the American Medical Association* 277, no. 12 (March 26, 1997): 985–89.

19. Young, *American Health Quackery*, 24–25; Francis D. Moore, "Therapeutic Innovation: Ethical Boundaries in the Initial Clinical Trials of New Drugs and Surgical Procedures," *Daedalus* 98, no. 2 (Spring 1969): 517–18.

20. Young, *American Health Quackery*, 24–25; Norman Gevitz, "Three Perspectives on Unorthodox Medicine," in *Other Healers: Unorthodox Medicine in America*, edited by Norman Gevitz (Baltimore: Johns Hopkins University Press, 1988), 17–18.

21. James C. Petersen and Gerald E. Markle, "Politics and Science in the Laetrile Controversy," *Social Studies of Science* 9, no. 2 (May 1979): 150, 154.

22. Michael S. Goldstein, *Alternative Health Care: Medicine, Miracle, or Mirage?* (Philadelphia: Temple University Press, 1999), 37.

23. Paul A. Offit, *Overkill: When Modern Medicine Goes Too Far* (New York: Harper, 2020), 205–12.

24. Ernst, *So-Called Alternative Medicine*, 127–89.

25. See, for example, Gisèle Chvetzoff and Ian F. Tannock, "Placebo Effects in Oncology," *Journal of the National Cancer Institute* 95, no. 1 (January 1, 2003): 19–29; Eric S. Zhou, Kathryn T. Hall, Alexis L. Michaud, Jaime L. Blackmon, Ann H. Partridge, and Christopher J. Recklitis, "Open-Label Placebo Reduces Fatigue in Cancer Survivors: A Randomized Trial," *Supportive Care in Cancer* 27 (2019): 2179–87. See also Offit, *Do You Believe in Magic?* chap. 11.

26. Offit, *Do You Believe in Magic?* epilogue.

27. Ernst, *So-Called Alternative Medicine*, 11; Harriet Hall, "'The Truth about Cancer' Series Is Untruthful about Cancer," *Science-Based Medicine*, November 17, 2015, https://sciencebasedmedicine.org/the-truth-about-cancer-series-is-untruthful-about-cancer/; Curt Devine and Drew Griffin, "Leaders of the Anti-vaccine Movement Used 'Stop the Steal' Crusade to Advance Their Own Conspiracy Theories," CNN.com, last updated February 5, 2021, https://www.cnn.com/2021/02/04/politics/anti-vaxxers-stop-the-steal-invs/index.html.

28. See, for example, Bernice L. Hausman, *Anti/Vax: Reframing the Vaccination Controversy* (Ithaca, NY: ILR, 2019); Frank Fischer, "Post-truth Populism and Scientific Expertise: Climate and Covid Policies from Trump to Biden," *International Review of Public Policy* 4, no. 1 (2022): 115–22, https://doi.org/10.4000/irpp.2390; Yasmeen Abutaleb, Rachel Roubein, and Isaac Arnsdorf, "For GOP Base, Battles over Coronavirus Vaccines, Closures Are Still Fiery," *Washington Post*, January 31, 2023, https://www.washingtonpost.com/politics/2023/01/31/gop-base-covid-mandate-battles/.

29. Nneka McGuire, "How the U. of I. Turned Its COVID Test into a Money Maker," ChicagoMag.com, February 22, 2022, https://www.chicagomag.com/chicago-magazine/march-2022/spit-equity/.

30. See, for example, Matthew C. Ehrlich, *Dangerous Ideas on Campus: Sex, Conspiracy, and Academic Freedom in the Age of JFK* (Urbana: University of Illinois Press, 2021); Michael V. Metz, *Radicals in the Heartland: The 1960s Student Protest Movement at the University of Illinois* (Urbana: University of Illinois Press, 2019); John K. Wilson, "Academic Freedom and Extramural Utterances: The Leo Koch and Steven Salaita Cases at the University of Illinois," *AAUP Journal of Academic Freedom* 6 (2015), https://www.aaup.org/JAF6/academic-freedom-and-extramural-utterances-leo-koch-and-steven-salaita-cases-university#.Xy7mu0l7lBy; Susan Saulny, "U. of Illinois Manipulated Admissions, Panel Finds," *New York Times*, August 6, 2009, https://www.nytimes.com/2009/08/07/education/07illinois.html.

31. See, for example, Susan Svrluga, "Conservatives Seek Control over Public Universities with State Bills," *Washington Post*, June 3, 2023, https://www.washingtonpost.com/education/2023/06/03/republicans-college-bills-dei-tenure/.

32. Vincent T. DeVita Jr. and Elizabeth DeVita-Raeburn, *The Death of Cancer* (New York: Sarah Crichton, 2015), 191.

33. Hongoltz-Hetling, *If It Sounds like a Quack*, chap. 6; Joshua Sharfstein, "Déjà Vu at the FDA," *Milbank Quarterly* 95, no. 2 (June 2017): 247. See also Sydney Lupkin, "Drugmakers Are Slow to Prove Medicines That Got a Fast Track to Market Really Work," NPR.org, July 22, 2022, https://www.npr.org/sections/health-shots/2022/07/22/1110830985/drugmakers-are-slow-to-prove-medicines-that-got-a-fast-track-to-market-really-wo; Pam Belluck, "Inside a Campaign to Get Medicare Coverage for a New Alzheimer's Drug," *New York Times*, April 6, 2022, https://www.nytimes.com/2022/04/06/health/aduhelm-alzheimers-medicare-patients.html; Pam Belluck, "New Experimental Therapy for

A.L.S. Approved in Canada," *New York Times*, June 13, 2022, https://www.nytimes .com/2022/06/13/health/als-treatment-albrioza.html.

34. See, for example, Ken Bensinger, "DeSantis, Aiming at a Favorite Foil, Wants to Roll Back Press Freedom," *New York Times*, February 10, 2023, https:// www.nytimes.com/2023/02/10/us/politics/ron-desantis-news-media.html; Victor Pickard, "Revitalizing America's News Deserts," *Progressive*, November 30, 2022, https://progressive.org/magazine/revitalizing-americas-news-deserts-pickard/.

35. Paul Farhi, "The Magazine Story That Made Elizabeth Holmes Famous Could Now Help Send Her to Prison," *Washington Post*, December 16, 2021, https://www.washingtonpost.com/lifestyle/media/elizabeth-holmes-fortune -cover-theranos/2021/12/15/f2332ed8-5841-11ec-a808-3197a22b19fa_story .html; Seth Mnookin, *The Panic Virus: A True Story of Medicine, Science, and Fear* (New York: Simon and Schuster, 2011), e-book, introduction; "National Survey Reveals Surprising Number of Americans Believe Alternative Thera- pies Can Cure Cancer," news release, October 30, 2018, American Society of Clinical Oncology, https://www.asco.org/news-initiatives/policy-news-analysis /national-survey-reveals-surprising-number-americans-believe.

36. John C. Burnham, "American Medicine's Golden Age: What Happened to It?," *Science* 215, no. 4539 (March 19, 1982): 1474.

37. John R. Thelin, *A History of American Higher Education*, 3rd ed. (Balti- more: Johns Hopkins University Press, 2019), e-book, chap. 7; Karin Fischer, "The Shrinking of Higher Ed," *Chronicle of Higher Education*, August 12, 2022, https://www.chronicle.com/article/the-shrinking-of-higher-ed.

38. Daniel C. Hallin, "The Passing of the 'High Modernism' of American Journalism Revisited," *Political Communication Report* 16, no. 1 (2005), https:// doczz.net/doc/8889460/the-passing-of-the-high-modernism-of-american.

39. Philip J. Hilts, *Protecting America's Health: The FDA, Business, and One Hundred Years of Regulation* (New York: Alfred A. Knopf, 2003), 144–65; Dan- iel Carpenter, *Reputation and Power: Organizational Image and Pharmaceutical Regulation at the FDA* (Princeton, NJ: Princeton University Press, 2010), 213–97; Jennifer Vanderbes, *Wonder Drug: The Secret History of Thalidomide in America and Its Hidden Victims* (New York: Random House, 2023).

40. Paul Starr, *The Social Transformation of American Medicine* (New York: Basic Books, 1982), 280–89.

41. Robert M. MacIver, *Academic Freedom in Our Time* (New York: Columbia University Press, 1955), 63. See also Ellen W. Schrecker, *No Ivory Tower: McCar- thyism and the Universities* (New York: Oxford University Press, 1986); Clark Kerr, *The Uses of the University*, 5th ed. (Cambridge, MA: Harvard University Press, 2001); Thelin, *History of American Higher Education*, e-book, chap. 7; John R. Thelin, *Going to College in the Sixties* (Baltimore: Johns Hopkins University Press, 2018), e-book, chap. 3.

42. Edwin R. Bayley, *Joe McCarthy and the Press* (Madison: University of Wis- consin Press, 1981); Edward Alwood, *Dark Days in the Newsroom: McCarthyism Aimed at the Press* (Philadelphia: Temple University Press, 2007).

43. James Harvey Young, *The Medical Messiahs: A Social History of Health Quackery in Twentieth-Century America* (Princeton, NJ: Princeton University Press, 1992), 406.

44. Young, *American Health Quackery*, 236–42; Herbert Bailey, *Real Hope to Cure Cancer* (New York: Feature Publications, 1960), John F. Kennedy Presidential Library and Museum Archives, Boston, MA, https://www.jfklibrary.org/asset-viewer/archives/JFKWHSFLCW/006/JFKWHSFLCW-006-009?image_identifier=JFKWHSFLCW-006-009-p0086.

45. Mukherjee, *Emperor of All Maladies*, 364–92; Sam Apple, *Ravenous: Otto Warburg, the Nazis, and the Search for the Cancer-Diet Connection* (New York: Liveright, 2021), e-book, chaps. 18–20; Charles Graeber, *The Breakthrough: Immunotherapy and the Race to Cure Cancer* (New York: Twelve, 2018); Michael S. Kinch, *The End of the Beginning: Cancer, Immunity, and the Future of a Cure* (New York: Pegasus, 2019); Jason Fung, *The Cancer Code: A Revolutionary New Understanding of a Medical Mystery* (New York: Harper Wave, 2020); Pickert, "Is a Revolution?"

46. Ellen Leopold, *A Darker Ribbon: Breast Cancer, Women, and Their Doctors in the Twentieth Century* (Boston: Beacon, 1999), 144–45.

47. Stoddard, *Krebiozen*, 5, 138–39; Young, *American Health Quackery*, 31.

48. Andrew Conway Ivy, interviewed and recorded by James David Boyle, November 4, 1968 (transcript), 21, National Library of Medicine, https://oculus.nlm.nih.gov/cgi/t/text/text-idx?c=oralhist;cc=oralhist;rgn=main;view=text;idno=2935142r; Bruno Klopfer, "Psychological Variables in Human Cancer," *Journal of Projective Techniques* 21, no. 4 (December 1957): 337–39.

Chapter 1. Substance X

1. *Illini Years: A Picture History of the University of Illinois* (Urbana: University of Illinois Press, 1950), 90, 100–101; American Council on Education, *University of Illinois: Survey Report by a Commission of the American Council on Education* (Washington, DC: American Council on Education, 1943), 70. See also David D. Henry, *Challenges Past, Challenges Present: An Analysis of American Higher Education since 1930* (San Francisco, CA: Jossey-Bass, 1975), 12–54.

2. George D. Stoddard, *The Pursuit of Education: An Autobiography* (New York: Vantage, 1981), 104. The university president who called the U of I a "sleeping giant" was James L. Morrill of the University of Minnesota (Winton U. Solberg and Robert W. Tomilson, "Academic McCarthyism and Keynesian Economics: The Bowen Controversy at the University of Illinois," *History of Political Economy* 29, no. 1 [1997]: 57).

3. Dudley McAllister, "Stoddard U.I. President July 1, 1946," *Sunday Courier* (Urbana, IL), May 27, 1945, 1, 3; "A New President," *Sunday Courier* (Urbana, IL), May 27, 1945, 6.

4. "1946," *Daily Illini*, January 3, 1946, 3.

5. Henry, *Challenges Past*, 55–68; John R. Thelin, *A History of American Higher Education*, 3rd ed. (Baltimore: Johns Hopkins University Press, 2019), e-book,

chap. 7; Glenn C. Altschuler and Stuart M. Blumin, *The GI Bill: A New Deal for Veterans* (New York: Oxford University Press, 2009), e-book, chap. 4.

6. "Student Enrollment Has 3440 Increase over Last Year," *Daily Illini*, November 18, 1945, 1; "UI Enrollment Is Second Largest," *Daily Illini*, March 14, 1947, 1; "Enrollment Up 6.12 Percent over Registration Last Fall," *Daily Illini*, October 10, 1947, 1; "Vet Enrollment for Semester Totals 10,834," *Daily Illini*, May 21, 1947, 2.

7. *Illini Years*, 113–14; Lex Tate and John Franch, *An Illini Place: Building the University of Illinois Campus* (Urbana: University of Illinois Press, 2017), 39; P. S. Ehrlich, *To Be Honest: Three Generations of Unexpectedly Dramatic Family Saga*, chap. 15, https://www.skeeterkitefly.com/tbhon_15.htm. See also Henry, *Challenges Past*, 62–65.

8. "Willard Issues Housing Appeal," *Daily Illini*, January 18, 1946, 1; "Five Cafes End Discrimination," *Daily Illini*, September 11, 1946, 1; Betty Duncan, "Parade Ground Councilmen to Govern, Publish Paper," *Daily Illini*, November 4, 1947, 1; Leslie J. Reagan, "Timothy Nugent: 'Wheelchair Students' and the Creation of the Most Accessible Campus in the World," in *The University of Illinois: Engine of Innovation*, edited by Frederick E. Hoxie, 50–59 (Urbana: University of Illinois Press, 2017).

9. "S-CIC Opens Fight against Theaters," *Daily Illini*, February 19, 1947, 1; "Interracial Committee Reports End of Pool Discrimination," *Daily Illini*, July 29, 1947, 1; Deirdre Lynn Cobb, "Race and Higher Education at the University of Illinois, 1945 to 1955" (PhD diss., University of Illinois at Urbana-Champaign, 1998); Altschuler and Blumin, *GI Bill*, chap. 5.

10. Paula S. Fass, *Outside In: Minorities and the Transformation of American Education* (New York: Oxford University Press, 1989), 164; Helen Farlow, "Dear Prexy: Please Teach Us Girls How to Earn Living," *Champaign-Urbana Courier*, c. July 1952, series 2/10/20, box 27, George D. Stoddard Papers, University of Illinois at Urbana-Champaign Archives; "UI's Dean Miriam Shelden Dies at 62," *News-Gazette* (Champaign, IL), May 13, 1975, sec. 1, 3; Eleanor Saunders Towns, interview by Anna Trammell, *Voices of Illinois Oral History Project*, May 22, 2018, https://www.library.illinois.edu/voices/collection-item/eleanor-saunders-towns/.

11. "Academic Life Begins at 40," *Decatur Herald* (IL), June 5, 1947, 6; Stoddard, *Pursuit of Education*, 112; Howard R. Bowen, *Academic Recollections* (New York: Macmillan, 1988), 26.

12. Stoddard, *Pursuit of Education*, 112–13, 122–23; *Illini Years*, 110, 114; Katie Buzard, "Public Broadcasting's Roots in Urbana," Illinois Public Media, June 2, 2022, https://will.illinois.edu/will100/story/will-the-naeb-and-public-broadcasting-as-we-know-it-today; Josh Shepperd, *Shadow of the New Deal: The Victory of Public Broadcasting* (Urbana: University of Illinois Press, 2023).

13. George D. Stoddard, "Stoddard's Achievement" (letter to the editor), *Chicago Tribune*, July 9, 1974, 10; Muriel Scheinman, "Celebrating Art: From Plaster Casts to Contemporary American Art Festivals," in *No Boundaries: University of Illinois Vignettes*, edited by Lillian Hoddeson, 304–13 (Urbana: University of Illinois Press, 2004); Bob Wilbert, "New Painting 'Represents a Trend,' Hard

to Understand: McKinney," *Daily Illini*, March 16, 1948, 1; "Professor Urges Revolt of Youth," *Daily Illini*, October 4, 1952, 2.

14. Ted Berland, "Invisible High-Energy X-Rays Being Used to Fight Cancer," *Daily Illini*, February 23, 1950, 1–2; "The Biggest Betatron in the World," *Life*, March 20, 1950, 129–32; Sylvian R. Ray, "The IILIACs and the Rise to Prominence in Computer Science," in *No Boundaries*, 226–40; Lillian Hoddeson, "John Bardeen: A Place to Win Two Nobel Prizes and Make a Hole in One," in *No Boundaries*, 241–58.

15. "Scientist's Scientist," *Time*, February 10, 1941, http://content.time.com /time/subscriber/article/0,33009,932565,00.html; "Man Television Machine, Italian Scientist Says," *Chicago Tribune*, November 27, 1934, 11.

16. Charles Leavelle, "Undergoes Test of How It Feels to Drop 7 Miles," *Chicago Tribune*, August 29, 1940, 3; "Tells of Need for Keeping Up Worker Health," *Chicago Tribune*, January 13, 1942, 24; "Appoint Dr. Ivy Navy's Medical Research Chief," *Chicago Tribune*, October 25, 1942, 19; "Lazy? No! You Just Don't Get the Right Diet," *Chicago Tribune*, July 8, 1943, 9; "War Scientists Create Drink of Sea Water," *Chicago Tribune*, April 12, 1944, 29; "N.U. Given $175,000 for Research on Infantile Paralysis," *Chicago Tribune*, June 21, 1944, 20; "N.U. Scientist's Discovery Aids War on Syphilis," *Chicago Tribune*, August 27, 1944, 14; "New Treatment for Alcoholics Started by City," *Chicago Tribune*, June 29, 1947, 30; "Dr. Ivy Offers 3 Point Plan to Curb Drug Evils," *Chicago Tribune*, February 3, 1950, B10; "Dr. Ivy Begins Self Defense," *Daily Illini*, December 2, 1965, 2; "'The Physiologist': A. C. Ivy, M.D.," *Ivy Cancer News*, November 1974, box 94, folder 11, A. C. Ivy Papers, American Heritage Center, University of Wyoming, Laramie [hereafter, Ivy Papers]; Warren R. Young, "What Ever Happened to Dr. Ivy?," *Life*, October 9, 1964, 114.

17. Leonard R. Temme, "Ethics in Human Experimentation: The Two Military Physicians Who Helped Develop the Nuremberg Code," *Aviation, Space, and Environmental Medicine* 74, no. 12 (December 2003): 1299; A. C. Ivy and Irwin Ross, *Religion and Race: Barriers to College?* (New York: Public Affairs Committee, 1949), 27; "Citizen Doctor," *Time*, January 13, 1947, https://content.time.com /time/subscriber/article/0,33009,855589,00.html. Although Ivy did help write the Nuremberg Code, the true extent of his contributions has been questioned (Paul Weindling, "The Origins of Informed Consent: The International Scientific Commission on Medical War Crimes, and the Nuremberg Code," *Bulletin of the History of Medicine* 75, no. 1 [Spring 2001]: 37–71; Allan Gaw, "Reality and Revisionism: New Evidence for Andrew C. Ivy's Claim to Authorship of the Nuremberg Code," *Journal of the Royal Society of Medicine* 107, no. 4 [2014]: 138–43).

18. Jon M. Harkness, "Nuremberg and the Issue of Wartime Experiments on US Prisoners," *Journal of the American Medical Association* 276, no. 20 (November 27, 1996): 1672–75; Carl Wiegman, "3 N.U. Officials Held Innocent," *Chicago Tribune*, June 29, 1945, 1.

19. Carl Wiegman, "$350,000 Being Spent by N.U. on Animal Labs," *Chicago Tribune*, June 22, 1945, 16; "Citizen Doctor," *Time*; Charles Leavelle, "Scientist Who's Always in a Hurry," *St. Louis Post-Dispatch*, April 4, 1947, 3D.

20. Patricia Spain Ward, "100 Years," *'Scope* 8, no. 3 (1981–82): 23–24.

21. Stoddard, *Pursuit of Education*, 111.

22. Thelin, *History of American Higher Education*, e-book, chap. 9; Winton U. Solberg, "Edmund Janes James," *American National Biography*, February 2000, https://doi.org/10.1093/anb/9780198606697.article.0900384.

23. Clark Kerr, *The Uses of the University*, 5th ed. (Cambridge, MA: Harvard University Press, 2001), 1–34. See also John R. Thelin, *Going to College in the Sixties* (Baltimore: Johns Hopkins University Press, 2018), e-book, chap. 3.

24. George D. Stoddard, "An Autobiography," *Yearbook of the National Society for the Study of Education* 70, no. 2 (1971): 331.

25. George D. Stoddard, *The Meaning of Intelligence* (New York: Macmillan, 1943), 33–34 (emphasis in original). See also Stoddard, *Pursuit of Education*, 51–66, 263–72.

26. "Catholic Bishop James A. Griffin, Springfield, Dies," *Decatur Daily Review* (IL), August 6, 1948, 1; Rev. John Evans, "Stoddard Assailed; Replies to Bishop," *Chicago Tribune*, October 1, 1945, 8; "Bishop Griffin Says Telegram from Stoddard 'Clears Atmosphere,'" *Freeport Journal-Standard*, October 20, 1945, 7.

27. Brad Dressler, "Russian People Desire Peace, AYD Hears," *Daily Illini*, May 22, 1946, 3; Jim Shacter, "6,500 Enthusiastically Greet Robeson's Delayed Concert; Singer Upholds AYD," *Daily Illini*, April 17, 1947, 1, 5.

28. "The Truth about AYD," *Daily Illini*, March 20, 1947, 1; "Clabaugh's AYD Bill Made Law by Governor," *Daily Illini*, August 9, 1947, 1. For more on the Clabaugh Act, see Matthew C. Ehrlich, *Dangerous Ideas on Campus: Sex, Conspiracy, and Academic Freedom in the Age of JFK* (Urbana: University of Illinois Press, 2021); Michael V. Metz, *Radicals in the Heartland: The 1960s Student Protest Movement at the University of Illinois* (Urbana: University of Illinois Press, 2019).

29. "Stoddard Speech Warns against Communism," *Daily Illini*, January 31, 1952, 1; Gar Fritts, "No Communists at University, Ewers Says," *Daily Illini*, September 30, 1950, 1, 3; Nicholas Wisseman, "Falsely Accused: Cold War Liberalism Reassessed," *Historian* 66, no. 2 (Summer 2004): 320–34.

30. Fritts, "No Communists," 3; Ellen W. Schrecker, *No Ivory Tower: McCarthyism and the Universities* (New York: Oxford University Press, 1986), 258; Wisseman, "Falsely Accused," 327–28; *Cold War: Illinois Stories*, Big Ten Network, 2021, https://www.youtube.com/watch?v=yhO4n7AOCcY.

31. Walter Gellhorn, ed., *The States and Subversion* (Ithaca, NY: Cornell University Press, 1952), 136; Wisseman, "Falsely Accused," 323, 329.

32. American Council on Education, *University of Illinois*, 7, 22; "Probe of U. of I. Medical School Reopens Today," *Chicago Tribune,* March 31, 1949, part 3, 19; "Dean Explains Resignation from UI," *Daily Illini*, November 17, 1949, 1; Ward, "100 Years," 24.

33. Howard E. Shuman, interview by Donald A. Ritchie, Oral History Project, United States Senate Historical Office, August 19, 1987, 218–19, https://www.senate.gov/about/resources/pdf/shuman-howard-e-full-transcript-with-index.pdf.

34. Eddie Jacquin, "Some Faculty Friends Are Troubled," *News-Gazette*, May 25, 1950, series 5/1/21, box 6, Coleman R. Griffith Papers, University of Illinois at Urbana-Champaign Archives [hereafter, Griffith Papers].

35. "The Legislature and Dr. Stoddard," *Chicago Tribune*, June 8, 1953, 16; Eddie Jacquin, "Time for Someone to Take Charge," *News-Gazette*, May 18, 1950, box 6, Griffith Papers. See also Stoddard, *Pursuit of Education*, 178–92.

36. "78.5 Million Still Should Be Enough for Great UI," *News-Gazette*, March 22, 1953, 4.

37. "UI Labor Institute Panel Advocates T-H Law Repeal," *Daily Illini*, December 10, 1948, 7; "House Appropriations Group May Oppose Budget: Dillavou," *Daily Illini*, May 28, 1949, 1; Marie Reno, "Peters Avers Some ILIR Employe[e]s Should Be Discharged for Activity," *Daily Illini*, July 13, 1949, 1; "Bradley's Resignation Accepted by University Trustees Board," *Daily Illini*, July 29, 1949, 1; Wisseman, "Falsely Accused," 332.

38. Details of the College of Commerce controversy come from Solberg and Tomilson, "Academic McCarthyism"; and Bowen, *Academic Recollections*, 25–35.

39. Bowen, *Academic Recollections*, 31; Solberg and Tomilson, "Academic McCarthyism," 72; "Economics at Illinois," *Chicago Tribune*, May 31, 1950, 20; "Deny Reds Rule U. of I. Faculty," *Chicago Herald-American*, June 23, 1950, box 6, Griffith Papers.

40. J. Neely Martin, "Downstate Bloc Names Grange for U.I. Race," *Decatur Herald* (IL), August 12, 1950, 3; Paula Peters, "'I'd Do It Again,' Says Stoddard," *Champaign-Urbana Courier*, October 26, 1969, 3; "Clabaugh Says Confidence in UI Shaken," October 6, 1950,, box 6, Griffith Papers.

41. Executive Committee of the College of Fine and Applied Arts, "Report on Conditions in the School of Music," June 27, 1950, box 6, Griffith Papers; Solberg and Tomilson, "Academic McCarthyism," 65; Bowen, *Academic Recollections*.

42. "Will There Always Be a Christmas?," *Daily Illini*, December 20, 1950, 8; George Thiem, "Expect Stoddard to Keep U.I. Helm," *Chicago Daily News*, December 29, 1950, box 6, Griffith Papers.

43. Jean Worth, "Bell and Gossett's Head Is Champion in Sales Game," *Escanaba Daily Press* (MI), April 25, 1958, 3; "Sworn Statement of Humberto Loretani," box 71, folder 3, Ivy Papers; "Board Plans Installation," *Los Angeles Times*, December 30, 1945, part 2, 3. "Kositerin" sometimes would be spelled "Cositerin."

44. "Sworn Statement of Humberto Loretani"; R. E. Moore to Nathan William MacChesney, April 26, 1949, series 3/17/1, box 79, folder 3, J. Roscoe Miller Papers, Northwestern University Archives, Evanston, IL; Whet Moser, "How Housing Discrimination Created the Idea of Whiteness," ChicagoMag.com, May 28, 2014, https://www.chicagomag.com/city-life/May-2014/The-Case-for-Reparations-and-the-Legacy-of-Discrimination-Against-Probationary-Whites-in-Chicago/.

45. Unsigned letter (probably by Carlos Tanturi) to University of Illinois, c. 1953, series 34/1/1, box 28, Legal Counsel's Office Subject File, University of

Illinois at Urbana-Champaign Archives. Sources indicate that Tanturi was at the meeting and that he was a visiting professor from Argentina ("Inter-American Notes," *Americas* 2, no. 3 [January 1946]: 380; Young, "What Ever Happened to Dr. Ivy?," 121).

46. Fred W. Fitz to J. Roscoe Miller, July 20, 1949, series 3/17/1, box 79, folder 3, J. Roscoe Miller Papers, Northwestern University Archives, Evanston, IL. Patient records of Northwestern's tests of Kositerin are in the same folder.

47. Unless otherwise noted, accounts of Ivy's initial experiences with Durovic and Krebiozen come from A. C. Ivy, "The Human Interest Aspects of the Story of Krebiozen as of May 1, 1951," box 9, folder 2, Ivy Papers; A. C. Ivy, *The History of Krebiozen*, c. 1953, box 11, folder 1, Ivy Papers; and Herbert Bailey, *A Matter of Life or Death: The Incredible Story of Krebiozen* (New York: Macfadden, 1964), 31–71.

48. Ivy, *History of Krebiozen*.

49. Siddhartha Mukherjee, *The Emperor of All Maladies: A Biography of Cancer* (New York: Scribner, 2011), 21–23; Frank E. Adair, "To Solve the Mysteries of Cancer," *New York Times Magazine*, April 21, 1946, 18.

50. A. C. Ivy, "Biology of Cancer," *Science* 106, no. 2759 (November 14, 1947): 456; Arthur Watson, "New Cancer Cure Hopes Stirred by Mystery Drug," *New York Sunday News*, April 8, 1951, 90–91; Irv Kupcinet, "Kup's Column," *Chicago Sun-Times*, April 16, 1948, 65; Roy Gibbons, "Cancer 'Cure' Story False, Dr. Ivy Says," *Chicago Tribune*, April 17, 1948, 11.

51. Leonard Keene Hirshberg, "The Dead Mending the Living," *Pittsburgh Sun-Telegraph*, July 30, 1944, American Weekly sec., 8; William L. Laurence, "Tomorrow You May Be Younger," *Ladies' Home Journal*, December 1945, 23; William J. Broad, "How a Star Times Reporter Got Paid by Government Agencies He Covered," *New York Times*, August 9, 2021, https://www.nytimes.com/2021/08/09/science/william-laurence-new-york-times.html; "Hormone Test on Cancer Tissue," *New York Times*, May 8, 1949, E11.

52. Bailey, *Matter of Life or Death*, 43.

53. A. C. Ivy, "Cancer Research: Reasons for Hope," address to the Second Annual Training School of the American Cancer Society, October 27, 1949, box 2, folder 13, Ivy Papers.

54. Humberto Loretani to R. E. Moore, February 16, 1950, box 4, folder 2, Ivy Papers.

55. Ivy, *History of Krebiozen*; Bailey, *Matter of Life or Death*, 51–54; "Marguerite, 61, Famed Chicago Modiste, Dies," *Chicago Tribune*, March 20, 1951, part 3, 9.

56. "Dr. John F. Pick," April 22, 1953, series 34/1/1, box 28, Legal Counsel's Office Subject File, University of Illinois at Urbana-Champaign Archives; "Rites Set for Surgeon John Pick," *Chicago Tribune*, October 14, 1978, sec. 1B, 26.

57. John F. Pick to A. C. Ivy, December 31, 1950, box 86, folder 3, Ivy Papers (emphasis in original).

58. Bailey, *Matter of Life or Death*, 49–50; Ivy, *History of Krebiozen*.

59. Jerry Sohl, "Says New Cancer Drug May Be Greatest Medical Discovery," *Pantagraph* (Bloomington, IL), April 8, 1951, 3; A. C. Ivy, John F. Pick, and W. F. P. Phillips, *Observations on Krebiozen in the Management of Cancer* (Chicago: Henry Regnery, 1956), 5.

60. George D. Stoddard, *"Krebiozen": The Great Cancer Mystery* (Boston: Beacon, 1955), 7.

61. "Judge J. S. Boyle, Helped Consolidation of Courts," *Chicago Tribune*, November 29, 1983, sec. 4, 6; Bailey, *Matter of Life or Death*, 68.

62. Ivy, "Human Interest Aspects of Krebiozen."

Chapter 2. Krebiozen Does Not Exist

1. Roy Gibbons, "U. of I. Reveals Cancer Control Drug," *Chicago Tribune*, March 27, 1951, 1, 9; A. C. Ivy, *Krebiozen: An Agent for the Treatment of Malignant Tumors*, March 1951, box 1, folder 6, George D. Stoddard Papers, University of Illinois–Chicago Archives; Norman DeNosaquo, "Memorandum for the File: 'Krebiozen' Meeting," March 28, 1951, box 443, folder 1, American Medical Association Historical Health Fraud and Alternative Medicine Collection, Chicago, IL.

2. Gibbons, "U. of I. Reveals," 1; Jerry Sohl, "Says New Drug May Be Greatest Medical Discovery," *Pantagraph* (Bloomington, IL), April 8, 1951, 3; Arthur J. Snider, "Why Durovic Insists on Keeping Cancer Drug Formula a Secret," *Chicago Daily News*, March 28, 1951, 14; "Did You Ever Pray for a Miracle?" (advertisement), *Pantagraph* (Bloomington, IL), April 10, 1951, 13.

3. L. Paul Ralph to Andrew C. Ivy, April 27, 1951, box 297, folder 9, Gloria Swanson Papers, Harry Ransom Center, University of Texas at Austin [hereafter, Swanson Papers]; Herbert Bailey, *A Matter of Life or Death: The Incredible Story of Krebiozen* (New York: Macfadden, 1964), 59–61, 73–76; "Cathcart Funeral on Wednesday," *Wyoming State Tribune*, March 4, 1969, 2.

4. A. C. Ivy, *The History of Krebiozen,* c. 1953, box 11, folder 1, A. C. Ivy Papers, American Heritage Center, University of Wyoming, Laramie [hereafter, Ivy Papers]; Greer Williams, "The Dilemma of Doctor Ivy," *Modern Hospital*, May 1952, 65–66; Arthur J. Snider, "Doctors Try to Curb Clamor over New Cancer Drug," *Chicago Daily News*, March 27, 1951, 8.

5. "Sign Bill to Let Dr. Durovic and His Family Stay in U. S.," *Chicago Tribune*, July 18, 1952, 2.

6. Keith Wheeler, "Dr. Durovic Stirs Up Whirlpool of Intrigue," *Chicago Sun-Times*, March 27, 1951, 15.

7. Clayton Kirkpatrick, "Durovic's Life Reveals War Ancestry," *Chicago Tribune*, November 16, 1951, 1, 5; Clayton Kirkpatrick, "Durovic Freed from Axis Cell by Queen's Aid," *Chicago Tribune*, November 17, 1951, 3; Clayton Kirkpatrick, "Durovic Tells of Success Won with Krebiozen," *Chicago Tribune*, November 18, 1951, 5; Clayton Kirkpatrick, "Durovic Brings Krebiozen Here; Amazes Dr. Ivy," *Chicago Tribune*, November 19, 1951, 8–9; Clayton Kirkpatrick, "Medical Storm Is Created by Durovic's Drug," *Chicago Tribune*, November 20, 1951, 6.

8. Joan Campbell, "A View from the Library," *'Scope* 8, no. 3 (1981–82): 41.

9. Roy Gibbons, "Public Warned Cancer Cure Is Yet in Future," *Chicago Tribune*, March 28, 1951, 6; Keith Wheeler, "Krebiozen Shipment a Mystery," *Chicago Sun-Times*, March 29, 1951, 3, 21; Roy Gibbons, "Finder Charges Bid to Exploit His Cancer Drug," *Chicago Tribune*, March 29, 1951, 6; Kirkpatrick, "Durovic Brings Krebiozen Here," 8–9.

10. Wheeler, "Dr. Durovic Stirs Up," 15; Gibbons, "Finder Charges Bid," 6.

11. Ivy, *History of Krebiozen*; George D. Stoddard, *"Krebiozen": The Great Cancer Mystery* (Boston: Beacon, 1955), 38–39; A. H. Fiske to Stevan Durovic, April 20, 1951, box 297, folder 9, Swanson Papers; Raymond M. Rice to Paul Douglas, December 19, 1963, box 1278, Paul H. Douglas Papers, Abakanowicz Research Center, Chicago History Museum, Chicago, IL. Abbott Laboratories in Chicago also approached Stevan Durovic about potentially obtaining rights to the drug (E. H. Volwiler to Stevan Durovic, March 26, 1951, box 297, folder 9, Swanson Papers).

12. Stoddard, *Krebiozen*, 32–40, 144–57.

13. Stoddard, *Krebiozen*, 39–40; "A Regular Meeting of the Krebiozen Research Foundation," June 26, 1951, series 34/1/1, box 28, Legal Counsel's Office Subject File, University of Illinois at Urbana-Champaign Archives.

14. Helen Farlow, "Krebiozen Bomb—Exploded Four Years Ago—Still Reverberating," *Champaign-Urbana Courier* (IL), March 27, 1955, 3; Lee Shassere, "5 Women Give Living Proof of Drug's Power," *Chicago Tribune*, March 27, 1951, part 1, 10; DeNosaquo, "Memorandum"; Harlan English to A. C. Ivy, April 27, 1951, box 82, folder 22, Ivy Papers; National Advisory Cancer Council quoted in Stoddard, *Krebiozen*, 227.

15. "An Editorial: Krebiozen," *Proceedings of the Institute of Medicine of Chicago* 18, no. 14 (May 15, 1951): 310.

16. "New Drug Used in Cancer Treatment" (unidentified clipping), c. April 1951, series 3/17/1, box 79, folder 3, J. Roscoe Miller Papers, Northwestern University Archives, Evanston, IL; Arthur Watson, "New Cancer Cure Hopes Stirred by Mystery Drug," *New York Sunday News*, April 8, 1951, 90–91.

17. Barry L. Beyerstein, "Why Bogus Therapies Often Seem to Work," *Quackwatch*, July 24, 2003, https://quackwatch.org/related/altbelief/. See also Harriet Hall, "No, No, No, NO! Testimonials Are Not Evidence!" *Skeptical Inquirer*, March 22, 2021, https://skepticalinquirer.org/exclusive/no-no-no-no -testimonials-are-not-evidence/.

18. Snider, "Why Durovic Insists," 14; DeNosaquo, "Memorandum"; Oliver Field, interview by Robert G. Porter, July 12, 1982, 50, *History of the U.S. Food and Drug Administration*, https://www.fda.gov/media/81489/download.

19. A. C. Ivy, "The Human Interest Aspects of the Story of Krebiozen as of May 1, 1951," box 9, folder 2, Ivy Papers.

20. James G. Burrow, *AMA: Voice of American Medicine* (Baltimore: Johns Hopkins University Press, 1963), 117, 121. See also Pope Brock, *Charlatan: America's Most Dangerous Huckster, the Man Who Pursued Him, and the Age of Flimflam* (New York: Crown, 2008); Bliss O. Halling, "Bureau of Investigation,"

in Morris Fishbein, *A History of the American Medical Association, 1847 to 1947* (Philadelphia: Saunders, 1947), 1034–38.

21. Milton Mayer, "The Rise and Fall of Dr. Fishbein," *Harper's Magazine*, November 1949, 76; Milton Mayer, "The Dogged Retreat of the Doctors," *Harper's Magazine*, December 1949, 27. See also Elton Rayack, *Professional Power and American Medicine: The Economics of the American Medical Association* (Cleveland, OH: World, 1967).

22. Mayer, "Dogged Retreat," 26; Morris Fishbein quoted in Patricia Spain Ward, "United States versus American Medical Association et al.: The Medical Antitrust Case of 1938–1943," *American Studies* 30, no. 2 (Fall 1989): 124, 144. See also Paul Starr, *The Social Transformation of American Medicine* (New York: Basic Books, 1982), 280–89; Mayer, "Rise and Fall," 76–85; American Medical Association, *Caring for the Country: A History and Celebration of the First 150 Years of the American Medical Association* (Chicago: American Medical Association, 1997).

23. "Re: Dr. William F. P. Phillips," February 3, 1950, box 438, folder 5, American Medical Association Historical Health Fraud and Alternative Medicine Collection, Chicago, IL.

24. Dr. Peter S. Y. Neskow affidavit, May 16, 1952, box 71, folder 4, Ivy Papers; Ivy, *History of Krebiozen*; Roy Gibbons, "A.M.A. Report to Weigh Merit of Cancer Drug," *Chicago Tribune*, July 11, 1951, 20. See also Roy Gibbons, "Cancer 'Cure' Story False, Dr. Ivy Says," *Chicago Tribune*, April 17, 1948, 11.

25. Franklin C. Bing to Andrew C. Ivy, June 29, 1951, and A. J. Carlson to A. C. Ivy, August 3, 1951, both in box 82, folder 17, Ivy Papers.

26. Franklin Bing to Andrew Ivy, August 1, 1951, in Stoddard, *Krebiozen*, 157–61.

27. A. C. Ivy to Franklin Bing, August 6, 1951, box 295, folder 2, Swanson Papers; Franklin Bing to Andrew C. Ivy, August 8, 1951, and August 21, 1951, both in box 82, folder 17, Ivy Papers.

28. C. P. Rhoads with a response by A. C. Ivy, "Krebiozen," *Science* 114, no. 2959 (September 14, 1951): 285–86; "Strip-Tease Therapeusis," *New England Journal of Medicine* 245, no. 10 (September 6, 1951): 382.

29. Ivy, *History of Krebiozen*.

30. "A Status Report on 'Krebiozen,'" *Journal of the American Medical Association* 147, no. 9 (October 27, 1951): 864–73.

31. James E. Hague, "A Cancer 'Cure' and Its Backer Found Wanting," *Washington Post*, November 18, 1951, B3; "Another Cancer Cure Flops," *Chicago Tribune*, October 27, 1951, 8.

32. Roy Gibbons, "A.M.A. Probers Ban Krebiozen Use in Cancer," *Chicago Tribune*, October 26, 1951, 1, 6; "Cancer Society Report Assails Drug Krebiozen," *Chicago Tribune*, October 27, 1951, part 1, 7; Roy Gibbons, "Doctor Group Hits Dr. Ivy," *Chicago Tribune*, November 14, 1951, 1, 14.

33. A. C. Ivy to George Stoddard, July 30, 1952, series 2/10/19, box 1, George D. Stoddard Krebiozen File, University of Illinois at Urbana-Champaign Archives

[hereafter, Stoddard Krebiozen File]; Stevan and Marko Durovic affidavit, June 7, 1952, box 71, folder 2, Ivy Papers.

34. Gibbons, "A.M.A. Probers," 6.

35. Coleman R. Griffith, "Informal Notes on My Direct Connections to the Krebiozen Affair," September 23, 1953, series 5/1/21, box 8, Coleman R. Griffith Papers, University of Illinois at Urbana-Champaign Archives.

36. Fran Myers, "Stoddard Gives Support to Ivy on Med Charge," *News-Gazette* (Champaign, IL), November 15, 1951, 3, 16.

37. Griffith, "Informal Notes"; "Medics Rebuke Stoddard for Support of Dr. Ivy," *Champaign-Urbana Courier*, December 10, 1951, series 2/10/20, box 27, George D. Stoddard Papers, University of Illinois at Urbana-Champaign Archives; Stoddard, *Krebiozen*, 52.

38. Warren Cole quoted in Bailey, *Matter of Life or Death*, 133–35.

39. "Trustees Meet; Olson Made New Dean," *Daily Illini*, February 17, 1950, 1; "Dean Explains Resignation from UI," *Daily Illini*, November 17, 1949, 1; Patricia Spain Ward, "'Who Will Bell the Cat?' Andrew C. Ivy and Krebiozen," *Bulletin of the History of Medicine* 58, no. 1 (Spring 1984): 35n21.

40. William G. Rothstein, *American Medical Schools and the Practice of Medicine: A History* (New York: Oxford University Press, 1987), 235–55; Roger L. Geiger, *American Higher Education since World War II: A History* (Princeton, NJ: Princeton University Press, 2019), 72–88; Clark Kerr, *The Uses of the University*, 5th ed. (Cambridge, MA: Harvard University Press, 2001), 35–63; John R. Thelin, *A History of American Higher Education*, 3rd ed. (Baltimore: Johns Hopkins University Press, 2019), e-book, chap. 7; John R. Thelin, *Going to College in the Sixties* (Baltimore: Johns Hopkins University Press, 2018), e-book, chap. 3.

41. "Ivy to Head New Science Clinic," *Daily Illini*, December 3, 1947, 5; Ward, "Who Will Bell the Cat?" 32–33. See also Starr, *Social Transformation*, 338–51.

42. Kerr, *Uses of the University*, 1–34.

43. Stanley Olson to George Stoddard, November 20, 1951, in Stoddard, *Krebiozen*, 164–66.

44. "Statement by Dr. Stoddard to Joint Legislative Commission," December 8, 1953, in Stoddard, *Krebiozen*, 254–56.

45. Andrew Ivy to Robert Johnson, October 21, 1952, in Stoddard, *Krebiozen*, 179–80.

46. *Report of the Research Validation Committee Appointed by President George D. Stoddard of the University of Illinois*, September 10, 1952, box 1, Stoddard Krebiozen File; J. G. Garland, "Report of a Case Treated with Krebiozen," c. July 1952, box 3, Stoddard Krebiozen File; S. P. Reimann and T. C. Pomeroy, "Preliminary Observations of 40 Treated Krebiozen Patients," July 16, 1952, box 3, Stoddard Krebiozen File; Ivy, *History of Krebiozen*.

47. *Report of the Research Validation Committee.*

48. *Report of the Research Validation Committee.*

49. Roy Gibbons, "Committee Reports on Cancer Drug Tested by Dr. Ivy," *Chicago Tribune*, September 20, 1952, 1, 6.

50. Andrew Ivy statement, September 24, 1952, in Stoddard, *Krebiozen*, 171–72; Warren H. Cole to Andrew C. Ivy, September 26, 1952, box 11, folder 10, Ivy Papers.

51. "Report by President Stoddard to Board of Trustees of University of Illinois," November 14, 1952, in Stoddard, *Krebiozen*, 185–86; Roy Gibbons, "Doctor Ponders Plea to Reveal Krebiozen Data," *Chicago Tribune*, September 21, 1952, 45; "Charges Plot to Bare Secret of Krebiozen," *Chicago Tribune*, September 28, 1952, 34.

52. Stanley Olson, "Statement Read to the Department Heads of the College of Medicine," September 30, 1952, box 1, Stoddard Krebiozen File; Griffith, "Informal Notes."

53. "Elect Ike and GOP Congress," *Chicago Herald-American*, October 27, 1952, 1; Tom Pelton, "Anti-abortion Movement Pioneer, Newspaperwoman Effie Alley, 95," *Chicago Tribune*, May 1, 1994, sec. 2, 8.

54. Effie Alley, "Krebiozen and Cancer: Woman's Story of New Drug," *Chicago Herald-American*, October 14, 1952, 1, 4; Effie Alley, "Lawyer Tells Cancer Fight," *Chicago Herald-American*, October 17, 1952, 1, 8. Alley's series ran in several issues of the *Herald-American* in October and November of 1952; copies are in box 2, Stoddard Krebiozen File. See also Bailey, *Matter of Life or Death*, 190–94.

55. "Dr. Ivy Gives His View on Series," *Chicago Herald-American*, October 20, 1952, 4.

56. Andrew Ivy draft letter to be signed by George Stoddard, October 10, 1952, and George Stoddard to Andrew Ivy, October 13, 1952, both in Stoddard, *Krebiozen*, 172–76.

57. At one point, Stevan Durovic was quoted in the press as saying that he would immediately disclose the information about Krebiozen (Roy Gibbons, "Doctor to Bare Basic Secrets of Cancer Drug," *Chicago Tribune*, October 3, 1952, 1).

58. Stevan Durovic to Andrew Ivy, October 21, 1952, Andrew Ivy to Robert Johnson, October 21, 1952, Stevan Durovic to Andrew Ivy, November 9, 1952, and Andrew Ivy to Robert Johnson, c. November 1952, all in Stoddard, *Krebiozen*, 178–83.

59. Effie Alley, "U. of I. Calls for Krebiozen Data," *Chicago Herald-American*, November 7, 1952, 7.

60. "Report by President Stoddard," 185–87.

61. Olson, "Statement."

62. "Report by President Stoddard," 187 (emphasis in original).

Chapter 3. Conspiracies and Circuses

1. Meeting minutes of the College of Medicine faculty, November 21, 1952, series 2/10/19, box 1, George D. Stoddard Krebiozen File, University of Illinois at Urbana-Champaign Archives [hereafter, Stoddard Krebiozen File]; "Medical Men

Back Stoddard in 'Knock-Down, Drag-Out' Session," *News-Gazette* (Champaign, IL), November 22, 1952, 3. See also Patricia Spain Ward, "'Who Will Bell the Cat?' Andrew C. Ivy and Krebiozen," *Bulletin of the History of Medicine* 58, no. 1 (Spring 1984): 37–39.

2. Frances B. Watkins to George D. Stoddard, November 17, 1952, and George D. Stoddard to Frances B. Watkins, November 19, 1952, both in box 1, Stoddard Krebiozen File; George D. Stoddard to Adlai E. Stevenson, November 24, 1952, box 2, Stoddard Krebiozen File.

3. "Report by President Stoddard to Board of Trustees," November 28, 1952, in George D. Stoddard, *"Krebiozen": The Great Cancer Mystery* (Boston: Beacon, 1955), 196–202; Coleman R. Griffith, "Informal Notes on My Direct Connections to the Krebiozen Affair," September 23, 1953, series 5/1/21, box 8, Coleman R. Griffith Papers, University of Illinois at Urbana-Champaign Archives [hereafter, Griffith Papers]; "Solons to Talk over Krebiozen; Inspect UI," *News-Gazette*, December 10, 1952, 3.

4. Arthur J. Snider, "Ivy May Quit U. of I. over Cancer Drug," *Chicago Daily News*, November 17, 1952, 1, 8; Christopher D. Green, "Psychology Strikes Out: Coleman R. Griffith and the Chicago Cubs," *History of Psychology* 6, no. 3 (2003): 267–83; Coleman R. Griffith to Andrew C. Ivy, November 25, 1952, and Coleman R. Griffith to Wayne A. Johnston, November 25, 1952, both in series 1/20/3, box 4, Wayne A. Johnston Papers, University of Illinois at Urbana-Champaign Archives.

5. "Statement by Dr. Ivy to President Stoddard for Transmittal to Board of Trustees," November 24, 1952, in Stoddard, *Krebiozen*, 196 (emphasis in original); "Durovic Cites Earlier Report on Krebiozen," *Champaign-Urbana Courier* (IL), November 22, 1952, 3.

6. "Promise Open Trustee Meet on Krebiozen," *News-Gazette*, November 24, 1952, 3; "Stoddard Ban on Krebiozen Work 'Blunder,'" *News-Gazette*, November 25, 1952, 3; Helen Farlow, "Legislators Rap 'Rebuke' to Ivy," *Champaign-Urbana Courier*, November 17, 1952, 3, 13; "Ivy 'Attacker' Will Answer to Legislature: Libonati," *News-Gazette*, November 23, 1952, 3; Roy Gibbons, "4 Legislators to Enter U. of I. Krebiozen Row," *Chicago Tribune*, November 27, 1952, A10.

7. Ed Borman, "Stoddard Recommends Ivy's Demotion to Trustees," *News-Gazette*, November 28, 1952, 3, 16; Helen Farlow, "Stoddard Asks Board to Demote Dr. A. C. Ivy," *Champaign-Urbana Courier*, November 28, 1952, 1, 3; "Charge Stoddard Used Hitler's 'Big Lie' Technique in Cancer Tiff," *Dispatch* (Moline, IL), November 29, 1952, 12; Ed Borman, "UI Trustees May Give Ivy Leave to Find Answer on Krebiozen Value," *News-Gazette*, November 29, 1952, 3, 16; Fran Myers, "Broadwalk Tattler," *News-Gazette*, November 30, 1952, 2, 35.

8. Roy Gibbons, "Adopts Policy of 'Hands Off' on Krebiozen," *Chicago Tribune*, December 13, 1952, 1; "Ivy 'Attacker' Will Answer," 3; Effie Alley, "New Krebiozen Results Bared," *Chicago Herald-American*, December 22, 1952, box 8, Griffith Papers.

9. "Krebiozen—Who Is Right?," *Daily Illini*, November 19, 1952, 4; "Politics Enters Evaluation of Krebiozen Controversy," *Daily Illini*, December 4, 1952, 4; "Dr. Ivy Should Ease U. of I.'s Dilemma over Krebiozen," *Chicago Daily News*, December 19, 1952, 16; "The Ground Rules," *Chicago Tribune*, December 14, 1952, 24.

10. "Resolution by Council of Chicago Medical Society," December 9, 1952, and "Statement by Executive Committee of College of Medicine to Committee to Visit Educational Institutions," December 5, 1952, both in Stoddard, *Krebiozen*, 202–5, 210.

11. "Report by Committee on Krebiozen to University of Illinois Senate," December 19, 1952, and "Report by Committee on Academic Freedom to University Senate," December 19, 1952, both in Stoddard, *Krebiozen*, 210–14; A. J. Carlson to Roger Adams, December 14, 1952, in series 15/5/23, box 40, Roger Adams Papers, University of Illinois at Urbana-Champaign Archives; American Association of University Professors, "Excerpts from the 1915 *Declaration of Principles on Academic Freedom and Tenure*" and "Excerpts from the 1940 *Statement of Principles on Academic Freedom and Tenure* with 1970 Interpretive Comments," in Matthew W. Finkin and Robert C. Post, *For the Common Good: Principles of American Academic Freedom* (New Haven, CT: Yale University Press, 2009), 173–74, 184. See also Stoddard, *Krebiozen*, 71–78; Henry Reichman, *Understanding Academic Freedom* (Baltimore: Johns Hopkins University Press, 2021), 26–53.

12. "Resolution by University Senate," December 19, 1952, in Stoddard, *Krebiozen*, 214–15; Clayton Kirkpatrick, "Trustees Give Leave to Ivy at His Request," *Chicago Tribune*, December 23, 1952, 1, 4; Helen Farlow, "Ivy Granted 6-Months Leave by U.I. Board," *Champaign-Urbana Courier*, December 22, 1952, 1, 3; "Libonati Will Seek More Power for U.I. Trustees," *Champaign-Urbana Courier*, December 23, 1952, 3. The trustees ended up tabling Nickell's redrafted resolution at a subsequent meeting ("U. of I. Trustees Refuse Plea to Praise Dr. Ivy," *Chicago Tribune*, February 24, 1953, 7).

13. "Statement of Dr. Andrew C. Ivy," December 22, 1952, and Andrew Ivy, "The Krebiozen Problem: A Reply to Certain Criticisms and Rumors," November 26, 1952, both in box 1, Stoddard Krebiozen File; "Statement by Dr. Ivy to Committee to Visit Educational Institutions," December 1952, in Stoddard, *Krebiozen*, 205–10.

14. Don C. Matchan, "The Great Ivy—and Krebiozen," *Herald of Health*, July 1958, 6.

15. "Scientific Discoveries" (advertisement), *Hickory Press* (NC), October 4, 1894, 6; "A Wonderful Discovery!" (advertisement), *People's Party Paper* (Atlanta, GA), September 20, 1895, 3, https://chroniclingamerica.loc.gov/lccn/sn83016235/1895-09-20/ed-1/seq-3.pdf.

16. Eric S. Juhnke, *Quacks and Crusaders: The Fabulous Careers of John Brinkley, Norman Baker, and Harry Hoxsey* (Lawrence: University Press of Kansas, 2002), 14, 37, 51. See also Philip J. Hilts, *Protecting America's Health: The FDA, Business, and One Hundred Years of Regulation* (New York: Alfred A. Knopf, 2003); James

Burrow, *AMA: Voice of American Medicine* (Baltimore: Johns Hopkins University Press, 1963); James Harvey Young, *The Medical Messiahs: A Social History of Health Quackery in Twentieth-Century America* (Princeton, NJ: Princeton University Press, 1992).

17. James Harvey Young and Richard E. McFayden, "The Koch Cancer Treatment," *Journal of the History of Medicine and Allied Sciences* 53, no. 3 (July 1998): 254–84; Juhnke, *Quacks and Crusaders*, 82.

18. Warren R. Young, "What Ever Happened to Dr. Ivy?," *Life*, October 9, 1964, 118, 121; A. C. Ivy to Frank E. Dingle, April 5, 1954, box 84, folder 24, A. C. Ivy Papers, American Heritage Center, University of Wyoming, Laramie [hereafter, Ivy Papers]. See also Francis D. Moore, "Therapeutic Innovation: Ethical Boundaries in the Initial Clinical Trials of New Drugs and Surgical Procedures," *Daedalus* 98, no. 2 (Spring 1969): 502–22.

19. James Harvey Young, *American Health Quackery: Collected Essays* (Princeton, NJ: Princeton University Press, 1992), 238–39; Susan Ives, "Monday's Monument: Louis Pasteur Statue, Chicago, IL," SusanIves.com, March 30, 2020, https://susanives.com/2020/03/30/mondays-monument-louis-pasteur-statue-chicago-il/. See also Young and McFayden, "Koch Cancer Treatment," 269.

20. Farlow, "Ivy Granted 6-Months Leave," 1. See also Paul H. Douglas, *In the Fullness of Time: The Memoirs of Paul H. Douglas* (New York: Harcourt Brace Jovanovich, 1972); "Charles J. Jenkins," *Chicago Tribune*, December 10, 1954, part 2, 8.

21. "Statement by President Stoddard," August 3, 1953, in Stoddard, *Krebiozen*, 242–43.

22. "Legislator Calls for Probe of U. of I. Medical School," *Clinton Daily Journal and Public* (IL), March 26, 1949, 1; Bob Lahey, "'Politics Is People'—Marzullo," *Elk Grove Herald* (IL), June 12, 1975, 14; Robert Benjamin, "Vito's Tale: A Ward to the Wise," *Chicago Tribune*, May 17, 1982, sec. 6, 8.

23. William J. Conway, "That Hat-Tipping Is Rough on Hats, but It Wins Votes," *Dispatch* (Moline, IL), December 27, 1957, 2; "Libonati Will Seek to Curb Stoddard's Power at U. I.," *Champaign-Urbana Courier*, December 19, 1952, series 2/10/20, box 28, George D. Stoddard Papers, University of Illinois at Urbana-Champaign Archives [hereafter, Stoddard Urbana Papers].

24. Joseph H. Kiefer, "Town and Gown in the '30s," *'Scope* 8, no. 3 (1981–82): 35. See also "Bloc in Chicago Is a G.O.P. Issue," *New York Times*, April 13, 1964, 15; "Former GOP Lawmaker, Coach Peter J. Miller, 81," *Chicago Tribune*, May 23, 1991, sec. 2, 9; O. T. Banton, "Halsted Street, Sen. Libonati and Krebiozen," *Champaign-Urbana Courier*, March 14, 1953, 3, 7; Conway, "That Hat-Tipping," 2; "Libonati Regrets," *Chicago Daily News*, June 13, 1963, 12.

25. Mike Royko, *Boss: Richard J. Daley of Chicago* (New York: Dutton, 1971), 61–67; "U.I. Krebiozen Probe Wanted by 'Fanatics,'" *Champaign-Urbana Courier*, March 1, 1953, 3; "Legislator Calls for Probe," 1.

26. Griffith, "Informal Notes"; Stoddard, *Krebiozen*, 80; "Statement by Dr. Ivy to Joint Legislative Committee: Excerpt," March 18, 1953, in Stoddard,

Krebiozen, 216–17; "The Response of Dr. Andrew C. Ivy to Those Present at the Testimonial Dinner Given for Him," February 23, 1959, folder 1, Andrew Ivy Biographical and Correspondence Collection, Roosevelt University Archives, Chicago, IL.

27. "Libonati Asks Investigation of U.I. Drug Fight," *Champaign-Urbana Courier*, January 13, 1953, 3; Johnson Kanady, "OK's State Probe of Krebiozen Dispute," *Chicago Tribune*, February 25, 1953, 1–2; John Justin Smith, "How Four Years Canceled Boyle As a Somebody," *Chicago Daily News*, November 22, 1952, 4; Ed Borman, "Reporter's Notebook," *News-Gazette*, March 22, 1953, 3. John Boyle eventually returned to power as head of the Cook County Circuit Court system ("Judge J. S. Boyle, Helped Consolidation of Courts," *Chicago Tribune*, November 29, 1983, sec. 4, 6).

28. "U.I. Krebiozen Probe," 3; "Krebiozen Probe Okayed by Senate," *Champaign-Urbana Courier*, March 4, 1953, 3; "Stoddard, Ivy to Testify in Krebiozen Quiz," *Chicago Tribune*, March 12, 1953, 11.

29. George Tagge, "Ivy Says A.M.A. Tried to Interfere with Cancer Drug," *Chicago Tribune*, March 19, 1953, 1, 18; Arthur J. Snider, "Krebiozen Battle Mystery Grows," *Chicago Daily News*, March 19, 1953, box 10, folder 5, Ivy Papers; "First Report by President Stoddard to Joint Legislative Committee," March 18, 1953, in Stoddard, *Krebiozen*, 217–21 (emphasis in original); John Dreiske, "The Krebiozen Hearings," *Chicago Sun-Times*, March 21, 1953, 12.

30. "Second Report by President Stoddard to Joint Legislative Committee," in Stoddard, *Krebiozen*, 221–28; Durward G. Hall to Moloye M. Sokitch, December 11, 1942, box 19, Stoddard Urbana Papers; Henry P. Leverich to Paul H. Douglas, September 14, 1953, series 34/1/1, box 28, Legal Counsel's Office Subject File, University of Illinois at Urbana-Champaign Archives [hereafter, Legal Counsel's File].

31. Stoddard, *Krebiozen*, 19–20; Jules Dubois to George D. Stoddard, June 19, 1953, box 28, Legal Counsel's File.

32. Enrico Fantoni, "Nuclear Island: The Secret Post–WWII Mega Lab Investigated," *Wired*, February 14, 2011, https://www.wired.co.uk/article/nuclear-island?page=all.

33. Unsigned letter to University of Illinois, c. 1953, box 28, Legal Counsel's File; "Second Report by President Stoddard," 228. The unsigned letter to the U of I probably was from Carlos Tanturi, who was present at Durovic's 1949 meeting with Northwestern University's medical dean.

34. "Is Krebiozen Only an Old Remedy for Hypertension?," *Champaign-Urbana Courier*, March 26, 1953, 3; Robert W. Sink, "NU Chapter of Durovic Saga Told," *Champaign-Urbana Courier*, April 6, 1953, 3, 12; Robert W. Sink, "Parable of the Potent Potion," *Champaign-Urbana Courier*, December 1, 1952, 6.

35. "Krebiozen," *Chicago Tribune*, March 27, 1954, 10; John Bartlow Martin, "What Those Politicians Do to You!" *Saturday Evening Post*, December 12, 1953, 90. See also "History of the *Courier*," June 1977, Champaign County

Historical Archives, Urbana, IL, https://archivescatalog.urbanafreelibrary.org/polaris/custom/repository/000400000149.pdf.

36. Percy Wood, "Plot Charged against Dr. Ivy on Krebiozen," *Chicago Tribune*, April 10, 1953, 1, 12; John F. Sembower to A. C. Ivy, January 22, 1953, box 100, folder 8, Ivy Papers.

37. Helen Farlow, "Navy Krebiozen Ban Told; Durovics Allege Threats," *Champaign-Urbana Courier*, April 10, 1953, 3, 16; Percy Wood, "Recordings Fail to Show Krebiozen Plot," *Chicago Tribune*, April 12, 1953, 1, 6.

38. Percy Wood, "7 Cancer Victims Silent Witnesses at Krebiozen Hearing," *Chicago Tribune*, April 11, 1953, 1; Percy Wood, "Threat to Dr. Ivy Denied," *Chicago Tribune*, May 10, 1953, 1; Ed Borman, "AMA 'Falsified' Its Report on Krebiozen: Ivy," *News-Gazette*, May 9, 1953, and "Ivy's Ouster Seen: Reporter," *News-Gazette*, April 24, 1953, both in box 28, Stoddard Urbana Papers. See also Henry A. Szujewski, "'Krebiozen' in Treatment of Cancer," *Journal of the American Medical Association* 148, no. 11 (March 15, 1952): 929–33.

39. Wood, "7 Cancer Victims," 1; "Quiet Days for Stoddard," *Champaign-Urbana Courier*, April 12, 1953, 28; Percy Wood, "Durovic Tells of Offering to Sell Krebiozen," *Chicago Tribune*, April 26, 1953, 1, 4; Ed Borman, "Air Krebiozen Business Deal," *News-Gazette*, May 8, 1953, 1, 24.

40. "Quiet Days for Stoddard," 28; "Illinois Faculty Members on Staff Here Back Stoddard," *Chicago Tribune*, May 15, 1953, A13.

41. Gar Fritts, "Trustees Discuss Commerce Rift," *Daily Illini*, May 19, 1951, 1; Edward C. Budd, "Economist Tells Why He Resigned" (letter to the editor), *Daily Illini*, July 28, 1951, 2; "'Home Grown' U.I. Ag Dean Asked," *Champaign-Urbana Courier*, March 14, 1952, box 27, Stoddard Urbana Papers; "Statement by President Stoddard," 245–46. See also Winton U. Solberg and Robert W. Tomilson, "Academic McCarthyism and Keynesian Economics: The Bowen Controversy at the University of Illinois," *History of Political Economy* 29, no. 1 (1997): 55–81.

42. "'Get Hearing Aid': Howe to Critic," *Daily Illini*, June 5, 1951, 1; "WILL Officials State Educational TV Should Supplement Commercial TV," *Daily Illini*, August 7, 1951, 1, 3; "IBA Denounces Educational TV at University," *Daily Illini*, April 24, 1953, 1; "Pier Asks Independence, Wants Own University," *Daily Illini*, July 3, 1953, 1–2.

43. "Cutler 'Ashamed' of UI until 'They Get Rid of That Crew,'" *News-Gazette*, May 20, 1953; Ed Borman, "Stoddard Rule, UI 'Pinkos' Attacked by Rep. Horsley," *News-Gazette*, May 28, 1953; "U.I., Horsley 'Embroyled' over Son's Low Grades," *Champaign-Urbana Courier*, June 26, 1953; Helen Farlow, "'Poor Public Relations' Back of State Audit of U.I. Books," *Champaign-Urbana Courier*, June 28, 1953; "Stratton Kills Bill on U. of I. Vice President," *Champaign-Urbana Courier*, July 18, 1953, all in boxes 28 and 29, Stoddard Urbana Papers.

44. George D. Stoddard, "Paranoids versus the People," June 13, 1953, series 2/10/802, box 4, George D. Stoddard Addresses and Publications, University of Illinois at Urbana-Champaign Archives.

45. John M. Carroll, *Red Grange and the Rise of Modern Football* (Urbana: University of Illinois Press, 1999), 193; "Grange Pledges to Drive 'Pinks' from UI; Backs Sports Palace," *Daily Illini*, November 11, 1950, 1; "Stoddard Ouster Might Aid Livingston as Candidate," *Champaign-Urbana Courier*, July 26, 1953, 1.

46. Carroll, *Red Grange*, 193; Stoddard, *Krebiozen*, 100–103; Ed Borman, "Red Grange Calls the Play: Ex-UI Football Star Introduces Motion for Confidence Vote," *News-Gazette*, July 25, 1953, 1, 7; Johnson Kanady, "Dr. Stoddard Quits U. of I. after a Vote of 'No Confidence,'" *Chicago Tribune*, July 26, 1953, 1, 12.

47. Borman, "Red Grange Calls the Play," 1, 7; "Aide Says Stratton Directed Campaign to Oust Stoddard," *News-Gazette*, July 25, 1953, 1; "Stoddard Ouster," 1; Fran Myers, "Broadwalk Tattler," *News-Gazette*, July 27, 1953, 2.

48. "Stoddard Ouster," 1; "Stoddard Fired to Aid Chances of Livingston," *Champaign-Urbana Courier*, July 28, 1953, 12; Kanady, "Dr. Stoddard," 1, 12. Park Livingston did run for US Senate in Illinois in 1954 but lost in the Republican primary.

49. Kanady, "Dr. Stoddard," 12; "Stoddard Rips Livingston for Ouster Vote," *Chicago Tribune*, July 30, 1953, 1; "Statement by President Stoddard," 246.

50. "18 Department Heads Attack Stoddard Vote," *Chicago Tribune*, July 29, 1953, 15; Helen Farlow, "Stoddards Hold Final 'President's Reception' for 1,000 Well-Wishers," *Champaign-Urbana Courier*, July 30, 1953, 3; Helen Farlow, "Johnston Cancels Board Walk-out," *Champaign-Urbana Courier*, September 24, 1953, 3; Stoddard, *Krebiozen*, 109–10; "Alumni Group Criticizes U.I. Board Action," *Champaign-Urbana Courier*, August 26, 1953, 3.

51. "Lloyd Morey Can Bring UI to Even Keel, End Tension," *News-Gazette*, July 26, 1953, 4; "Termites in Urbana: Politicians Finally Liquidated Stoddard," *Chicago Sun-Times*, July 29, 1953, 23; "Stoddard Out," *Chicago Daily News*, July 27, 1953, 6; "Intrigue in Illinois," *St. Louis Post-Dispatch*, July 28, 1953, 2B; "Crime and Punishment," *Daily Illini*, July 28, 1953, 6.

52. "U.I. Trustees Still Have Responsibility," *Champaign-Urbana Courier*, July 27, 1953, 6.

53. Helen Farlow, "Attorney Charges No Horses Used in Making Krebiozen," *Champaign-Urbana Courier*, October 20, 1953, 3, 10; Helen Farlow, "Dr. Ivy Says Livingston Aided Krebiozen Parley," *Champaign-Urbana Courier*, October 7, 1953, 12; Helen Farlow, "Probe Krebiozen Publicity Meeting," *Champaign-Urbana Courier*, October 8, 1953, 3, 12; Percy Wood, "Ivy 'Rebuked' Drug Founder, Hearing Told," *Chicago Tribune*, October 8, 1953, 4; Stoddard, *Krebiozen*, 98–99.

54. Percy Wood, "2 Drugs Aren't Same, Durovic Shouts in Huff," *Chicago Tribune*, September 19, 1953, 18; Helen Farlow, "250,000 Glass Ampules Can't Be Located," *Champaign-Urbana Courier*, December 3, 1953, 3, 20.

55. Helen Farlow, "Cositerin Termed Versatile Cure-all," *Champaign-Urbana Courier*, November 4, 1953, 3, 12; Percy Wood, "Denies Claims of Dr. Durovic," *Chicago Tribune*, November 5, 1953, 1, 12; Percy Wood, "Witness Denies Seeking 2½ Million for Durovic Drugs," *Chicago Tribune*, November 6, 1953, 6.

56. Percy Wood, "Stoddard Criticizes Ivy in Krebiozen Row," *Chicago Tribune*, December 9, 1953, C6; "First Krebiozen Story Surprised U. of I. Administration: Stoddard," *Champaign-Urbana Courier*, December 9, 1953, 3, 12; Oliver Field, interview by Robert G. Porter, July 12, 1982, *History of the U.S. Food and Drug Administration*, 52, https://www.fda.gov/media/81489/download. See also Stoddard, *Krebiozen*, 111–16, 251–68.

57. Helen Farlow, "Krebiozen Hearing to Go On and On," *Champaign-Urbana Courier*, December 6, 1953, 3; Arthur J. Snider, "Hint Krebiozen Quiz to Collapse," *Chicago Daily News*, December 11, 1953, box 8, Griffith Papers; "73 of 76 Persons Treated with Krebiozen Now Dead," *Champaign-Urbana Courier*, March 11, 1954, 3; Johnson Kanady, "Legislative Probe Clears Ivy," *Chicago Tribune*, March 25, 1954, 1–2; "Preliminary Report of Joint Legislative Commission," March 24, 1954, in Stoddard, *Krebiozen*, 271–74. See also "Statement by American Medical Association to Joint Legislative Commission," c. March 1954, in Stoddard, *Krebiozen*, 268–71.

58. "Preliminary Report," 271–74; Kanady, "Legislative Probe Clears Ivy," 1–2; Helen Farlow, "'Details' Hold Up Settlement on Krebiozen," *Champaign-Urbana Courier*, December 12, 1953, 3, 9; "UI Rejects Ivy Proposal for Study of Drug," *News-Gazette*, December 31, 1953, box 8, Griffith Papers; "U. of I. out of Krebiozen Row," *Chicago Tribune*, March 7, 1954, 1.

Chapter 4. A Fair Test

1. Helen Farlow, "Krebiozen Seen 'Trigger' Touching Off Ouster Blast for President Stoddard," *Champaign-Urbana Courier* (IL), July 26, 1953, 3; George D. Stoddard, "Notes for a Seven-Year Report of the President of the University of Illinois, 1946–1953," and George D. Stoddard to Coleman and Louise Griffith, August 28, 1953, both in series 5/1/21, box 8, Coleman R. Griffith Papers, University of Illinois at Urbana-Champaign Archives.

2. Stoddard to Griffith; George D. Stoddard, *The Pursuit of Education: An Autobiography* (New York: Vantage, 1981), 199; "Stoddard Blasts Stratton Regime," *Champaign-Urbana Courier*, January 9, 1954, 3. For more on David Henry's U of I presidency and his relationships with the governor and trustees, see Matthew C. Ehrlich, *Dangerous Ideas on Campus: Sex, Conspiracy, and Academic Freedom in the Age of JFK* (Urbana: University of Illinois Press, 2021).

3. Stoddard, *Pursuit of Education*, 161, 199; George D. Stoddard to Eugene Reynal, February 28, 1954, series 002/01/01, box 3, folder 20, George Stoddard Papers, University of Illinois–Chicago Archives [hereafter, Stoddard Chicago Papers]. Details of Stoddard's advance from Harcourt, Brace and Company are in the same folder.

4. Stoddard, *Pursuit of Education*, 153–54; Eugene Reynal to George Stoddard, April 8, 1954, and George D. Stoddard to Willard B. Spalding, May 2, 1954, both in box 3, folder 20, Stoddard Chicago Papers; George D. Stoddard to Jeannette Hopkins, March 12, 1955, box 5, folder 39, Stoddard Chicago Papers.

5. George D. Stoddard, *"Krebiozen": The Great Cancer Mystery* (Boston: Beacon, 1955), 41, 55–56, 115, 123, 133. See also Rev. John Evans, "Sheil School Fetes Bishop; 2 Get Awards," *Chicago Tribune*, May 1, 1953, 10.

6. Correspondence between John F. Sembower and A. C. Ivy, March–May 1955, correspondence between John F. Sembower and John F. LeVinnes Jr., April 1955, and personal statements of A. C. Ivy, May 31, 1956, and March 27, 1961, all in box 68, folders 5–6, A. C. Ivy Papers, American Heritage Center, University of Wyoming, Laramie [hereafter, Ivy Papers].

7. Stoddard, *Pursuit of Education*, 170–72; "Halt Stoddard's 'Exposé' of Krebiozen," *Chicago Tribune*, April 8, 1955, 1; "Boston Attacks Press Freedom," *Chicago Tribune*, April 11, 1955, 18; "Reverses Rule Banning Book on Krebiozen," *Chicago Tribune*, July 8, 1955, 16; "$360,000 in Libel Asked by Ivy from Stoddard," *Chicago Tribune*, July 31, 1955, 18; "The Book They Couldn't Ban," box 438, folder 11, American Medical Association Historical Health Fraud and Alternative Medicine Collection, Chicago, IL [hereafter, AMA Collection].

8. "Herb Bailey Promotion Chief of New Radio Station WCON," *Atlanta Constitution*, November 8, 1947, 10; "Notes of the Theater," *Chicago Tribune*, January 26, 1947, part 6, 5; Carlton Fredericks and Herbert Bailey, *Food Facts and Fallacies: The Intelligent Person's Guide to Nutrition and Health* (New York: Julian, 1965), 381.

9. Herb Bailey, "How to Keep from Getting False Teeth," *Better Homes and Gardens*, November 1951, 32–36, 198–99; Herb Bailey, "Ultrasound: Industry's Vibration Gun," *Science Digest*, December 1950, 86–88; Herb Bailey, "Into the Mysteries of the Brain," *Collier's*, June 24, 1950, 34, 71–72; Herb Bailey, "Tell-Tale Hands," *Science Digest*, February 1951, 63–65.

10. "Pioneer in X-Ray Honored," *Decatur Daily Review* (IL), July 11, 1951, 3; Fredericks and Bailey, *Food Facts and Fallacies*, 381; Paul C. Hodges, *The Life and Times of Emil H. Grubbe* (Chicago: University of Chicago Press, 1964), vii; Herbert Bailey, *K, Krebiozen—Key to Cancer?* (New York: Hermitage House, 1955), 8.

11. Bailey, *K*, 9; Helen Farlow, "Ivy Granted 6-Months Leave by U.I. Board," *Champaign-Urbana Courier*, December 22, 1952, 1; "Stoddard Book on Krebiozen Set for March," *Champaign-Urbana Courier*, February 2, 1955, 3; Herbert Bailey, *Real Hope to Cure Cancer* (New York: Feature Publications, 1960), 25, John F. Kennedy Presidential Library and Museum Archives, Boston, MA [hereafter, JFK Archives], https://www.jfklibrary.org/asset-viewer /archives/JFKWHSFLCW/006/JFKWHSFLCW-006-009?image_identifier =JFKWHSFLCW-006-009-p0099; *False Witness*, c. 1953, JFK Archives, https://www.jfklibrary.org/asset-viewer/archives/JFKWHSFLCW/006 /JFKWHSFLCW-006-010?image_identifier=JFKWHSFLCW-006-010-p0002. See also Stoddard, *"Krebiozen,"* 61.

12. Drew Pearson, "Controversial Krebiozen Sent to Taft by Tobey," *Daily Illini*, August 5, 1953, 4; Benedict Fitzgerald report and addendum, c. 1953, box 8, folder 1, Ivy Papers; "Some Who Use Krebiozen Pay $9 an Ampule," *Chicago*

Tribune, June 24, 1954, 3. See also Donald A. Ritchie, *The Columnist: Leaks, Lies, and Libel in Drew Pearson's Washington* (New York: Oxford University Press, 2021).

13. Bailey, *K*; Herbert Bailey, *A Matter of Life or Death: The Incredible Story of Krebiozen* (New York: Macfadden, 1964); Herbert Bailey to Mel Arnold, March 24, 1955, box 298, folder 3, Gloria Swanson Papers, Harry Ransom Center, University of Texas at Austin [hereafter, Swanson Papers].

14. Bailey, *K*, vi; Herbert Bailey author statement, March 7, 1955, box 82, folder 14, Ivy Papers. Paul Muni starred in the 1937 movie *The Life of Emile Zola*. See also Adam Gopnik, "Trial of the Century," *New Yorker*, September 28, 2009, https://www.newyorker.com/magazine/2009/09/28/trial-of-the-century.

15. Bailey, *K*, 67–68.

16. Bailey, *K*, 120 (emphasis in original); Barbara Yuncker, "Krebiozen vs. Cancer: The Role of the AMA," *New York Post Daily Magazine*, September 28, 1960, 41. See also Bailey, *Matter of Life or Death*, 194–97.

17. Bailey, *K*, 184, 199.

18. Bailey, *K*, 198, 200–201.

19. "Statement by Cole Committee," June 24, 1953, in Stoddard, *Krebiozen*, 235–37.

20. Oliver Field to William A. Hyland, November 20, 1958, box 439, folder 7, AMA Collection.

21. Bailey, *Matter of Life or Death*, 183–84, 260–66; Gopnik, "Trial of the Century."

22. Bailey, *K*, 110–12, 144, 200, 226–27, 269–82 (emphasis in original); Bailey to Arnold; George D. Stoddard to Janet Finnie, March 12, 1955, box 5, folder 39, Stoddard Chicago Papers; Stoddard, *Pursuit of Education*, 172.

23. Bailey author statement (emphasis in original).

24. Wade Jones, *America's Incredible Cancer Case*, February 1955, box G229, folder 2, Drew Pearson Papers, Lyndon B. Johnson Presidential Library, Austin, TX [hereafter, Pearson Papers].

25. Jones, *America's Incredible Cancer Case*; Wade Jones to Jack Anderson, December 12, 1956, box G229, folder 1, Pearson Papers; Drew Pearson, "Washington Merry-Go-Round," *Montgomery Advertiser* (AL), November 25, 1956, B3.

26. A. C. Ivy, John F. Pick, and W. F. P. Phillips, *Observations on Krebiozen in the Management of Cancer* (Chicago: Henry Regnery, 1956), 75–84 (emphasis in original).

27. Revilo P. Oliver, "Observations on Krebiozen in the Management of Cancer," review of *Observations on Krebiozen* by A. C. Ivy, John F. Pick, and W. F. P. Phillips, *National Review*, November 24, 1956, 21; "Plans Complete for Testimonial Dinner February 23," *Ivy Cancer News*, February 1968, box 445, folder 8, AMA Collection. See also "About Regnery Publishing," https://www.regnery.com/our-story/; Ehrlich, *Dangerous Ideas on Campus*; Ritchie, *The Columnist*.

28. David M. Kasson, "A Cancer Patient Speaks: 'I Will Not Donate to the American Cancer Society,'" May 1957, box G229, folder 1, Pearson Papers; David M. Kasson, "How I Was Brought Back from the Dead," *Inside Story*, October 1957, box 3, folder 20, Stoddard Chicago Papers.

29. Kasson, "Cancer Patient Speaks"; "Committee for Independent Cancer Research," American Medical Association investigative memo, January 28, 1957, box 444, folder 11, AMA Collection; Gloria Swanson, *Swanson on Swanson* (New York: Random House, 1980), 314–17, 473–74, 511–14; Gloria Swanson to F. Allen Rutherford, August 6, 1960, box 299, folder 9, Swanson Papers.

30. *This Is Your Life* script, c. January 1957, box 157, folder 9, Swanson Papers; "Famed Actress Says She Fights for Truth," *Lebanon Daily News* (PA), September 15, 1958, 1, 18; "Gloria Swanson: 1957 TV Interview with Mike Wallace," *YouTube*, posted by Reel Old Movies, https://www.youtube.com/watch?v=AOq _i5htqO4. Letters responding to Swanson's television appearances on behalf of Krebiozen are in boxes 287–90 in the Swanson Papers.

31. Bailey, *Matter of Life or Death*, 305; Kasson, "Cancer Patient Speaks"; "Famed Actress Says She Fights for Truth," 1, 18; "Ivy Lecture Touches Off Test Campaign," *Lebanon Daily News*, September 15, 1958, 1, 18; William D. Morain, "Krebiozen: Nineteen Years of Controversy," talk presented at Harvard University, March 18, 1968, box 446, folder 2, AMA Collection. The ICRF eventually changed its name once more, becoming the Independent Citizens Research Foundation to indicate that it concerned itself with more than just cancer.

32. Allen Rutherford to Gloria Swanson, October 3, 1958, Allen F. Rutherford to Krebiozen Research Foundation, c. 1958, and Mignon Rutherford to Gloria Swanson, March 9, 1959, all in box 299, folder 9, Swanson Papers.

33. *A Matter of Life or Death* publicity release, c. 1958, box 299, folder 11, Swanson Papers; "Famed Actress Says She Fights for Truth," 1, 18; Edward T. Windham and Clarence Lyons to Vance Hartke, April 10, 1963, box 3609, Records of the Food and Drug Administration, National Archives and Records Administration, College Park, MD; "Labor Leader Urges New Test for Controversial Drug," *Pantagraph* (Bloomington, IL), March 5, 1959, 2; "Krebiozen on March!" *Chicago's American*, May 4, 1960, Record Group 016/01/01/20/04/01, box 1, folder 2, Granville Bennett Papers, University of Illinois–Chicago Archives; "State of Indiana Labor," *Ivy Cancer News*, October-November-December 1961, box 94, folder 11, Ivy Papers.

34. Percy Wood, "Ivy Announces Fund Drive to Aid Krebiozen," *Chicago Tribune*, February 24, 1959, A4; Program for Testimonial Dinner for Andrew Conway Ivy, February 23, 1959, box 295, folder 7, Swanson Papers.

35. William Leonard, "What about Krebiozen?," *Chicago Tribune*, May 10, 1959, G18–20; "Dr. Durovic Bares Krebiozen Loss," *Chicago Daily News*, April 13, 1959, 11; A. C. Ivy to Paul H. Douglas, July 5, 1960, Paul Douglas Papers, box 306, Abakanowicz Research Center, Chicago History Museum [hereafter, Douglas Papers].

36. Ivy Cancer Research Foundation promotional flyer, c. 1960, box 443, folder 5, AMA Collection; Leonard, "What about Krebiozen?," G18–20;

A. C. Ivy, George E. Park, and W. C. Dolowy, "Therapeutic Improvement of Canine Cataract," *Veterinary Medicine* 54, no. 4 (April 1959): 205–13.

37. Ivy to Douglas, July 5, 1960; Dorothea Seeber to Gloria Swanson, c. November 1959, box 295, folder 6, Swanson Papers.

38. Ivy to Douglas, July 5, 1960; "John M. Davis Funeral to Be Held Thursday," *Chicago Tribune*, June 22, 1960, part 3, 9; Barbara Yuncker, "Krebiozen vs. Cancer—Proposal for a Final Test," *New York Post Daily Magazine*, September 30, 1960, 21; Ralph Buntyn, "Meet the Boykos: A Family of Achievers," October 26, 2021, UnitedIsraelWorldUnion.com, https://unitedisraelworldunion .com/meet-the-boykos-a-family-of-achievers/; "A Statement of Purpose," *Bulletin of Citizens Emergency Committee for Krebiozen*, June 1960, box 296, folder 5, Swanson Papers; Bailey, *Real Hope to Cure Cancer*, 17, https://www.jfklibrary.org /asset-viewer/archives/JFKWHSFLCW/006/JFKWHSFLCW-006-009?image _identifier=JFKWHSFLCW-006-009-p0095. See also ad for Herbert Bailey's *Matter of Life or Death* in the *New York Times*, August 10, 1959, 15.

39. Barbara Yuncker, "The Krebiozen Drug: Does It Work against Cancer?," *New York Post Daily Magazine*, September 27, 1960, 29; Barbara Yuncker, "Krebiozen vs. Cancer: The Sideshows," *New York Post Daily Magazine*, October 2, 1960, 5; Yuncker, "Krebiozen vs. Cancer—Proposal for a Final Test," 21; "Krebiozen Plan Offered," *Chicago Daily News*, March 2, 1959, 3; "Krebiozen Again," *Chicago Tribune*, May 22, 1959, 10.

40. A. C. Ivy to Paul H. Douglas, March 6, 1959, box 312, Douglas Papers; Yuncker, "Krebiozen vs. Cancer—Proposal for a Final Test," 21. See also Perri Klass, "How Science Conquered Diphtheria, the Plague among Children," *Smithsonian Magazine*, October 2021, https://www.smithsonianmag.com/science -nature/science-diphtheria-plague-among-children-180978572/.

41. Ivy to Douglas, March 6, 1959; Jack Anderson to Drew Pearson, August 11, 1953, box G229, folder 2, Pearson Papers; Barbara Yuncker, "Krebiozen vs. Cancer: The Case Histories," *New York Post Daily Magazine*, September 29, 1960, 23.

42. Percy Wood, "Cancer Test of Krebiozen Is Discussed," *Chicago Tribune*, April 9, 1958, 26.

43. Percy Wood, "Fears Ivy Plan for Krebiozen Test Is Doomed," *Chicago Tribune*, June 27, 1958, 16; "Offer by Cancer Society Tests Krebiozen Backers," *Chicago Daily News*, March 11, 1959, box 443, folder 4, AMA Collection; John F. Allen, "Ex-Cancer Expert at Hearing Here," *San Francisco Examiner*, May 8, 1958, 15; John F. Allen, "Death Hastened by Cancer 'Cure' Pill, Probe Told; 2nd Drug Also Attacked," *San Francisco Examiner*, May 9, 1958, 15; "Ivy Questions Findings of 2 on Krebiozen," *Chicago Tribune*, June 22, 1958, 18.

44. Paul H. Douglas, "A Proposal for an Impartial Test of Krebiozen as a Cure for Cancer," August 22, 1958, box 1278, Douglas Papers; "Asks Meeting to Set Up Test of Krebiozen," *Chicago Tribune*, August 31, 1958, 11.

45. Zelma Lee Ross to Richard M. Stanley, November 26, 1958, and Prairie State Health Federation promotional materials, c. 1958, both in box 439, folder 7, AMA Collection; "The Krebiozen Battle," Independent Cancer Research

Foundation, fall 1959, box 291, folder 10, Swanson Papers; "U.S. Aid Urges More Studies of Krebiozen," *Chicago Tribune*, September 25, 1958, B10; "Douglas Seeks Cancer Tests for Krebiozen," *Chicago Tribune*, December 6, 1958, 13.

46. "Cancer Group Rejects Test of Krebiozen," *Chicago Tribune*, March 5, 1959, A9; American Cancer Society, "A Background Paper on Krebiozen," *Journal of the American Medical Association* 169, no. 15 (April 11, 1959): 1797.

47. Roy Gibbons, "Blast Cancer Society over Krebiozen Snub," *Chicago Tribune*, May 19, 1959, A1; Harold S. Diehl to Paul H. Douglas, June 19, 1959, box 312, Douglas Papers.

48. Percy Wood, "Hope National Cancer Institute Tests Krebiozen," *Chicago Tribune*, February 12, 1961, 9; Roy Gibbons, "New Batches of Krebiozen Called 'Safe,'" *Chicago Tribune*, October 4, 1960, 8; Bailey, *Real Hope to Cure Cancer*, 32–33, https://www.jfklibrary.org/asset-viewer/archives/JFKWHSFLCW/006/JFKWHSFLCW-006-009?image_identifier=JFKWHSFLCW-006-009-p0103; Yuncker, "Krebiozen vs. Cancer: The Role of the AMA," 41.

49. Stoddard, *Pursuit of Education*, 172–73; "Ivy Prepared to Put 200 on Stand at Trial," *Chicago Tribune*, April 5, 1961, 3; "Libel Jury to Decide on Worth of Krebiozen," *Chicago Tribune*, April 4, 1961, 1.

50. Julius H. Miner to Abraham A. Ribicoff, April 12, 1961, JFK Archives, https://www.jfklibrary.org/asset-viewer/archives/JFKWHSFLCW/006/JFKWHSFLCW-006-009?image_identifier=JFKWHSFLCW-006-009-p0052; "U.S. Approves Official Test of Krebiozen," *Chicago Tribune*, April 20, 1961, A6.

Chapter 5. Nothing but Creatine

1. "Proposal of Dean's Advisory Committee with Respect to Department of Clinical Science," May 9, 1960, Record Group 016/01/01/20/04/01, box 1, folder 5, Granville Bennett Papers, University of Illinois–Chicago Archives; "Act to Close Ivy Clinical Unit at U. of I.," *Chicago Tribune*, June 8, 1961, A4.

2. "Act to Close," A4; clippings, correspondence, and memos, June 1961–August 1961, series 2/15/10, box 3, Administrative and Personnel Actions File, University of Illinois at Urbana-Champaign Archives [hereafter, Administrative and Personnel Actions File]; "An Outrageous Intrusion," *Chicago Daily News*, June 8, 1961, 16; "U. of I. to Give Dr. Ivy Facilities for Research," *Chicago Tribune*, September 29, 1961, A13.

3. Roland V. Libonati to David D. Henry, July 20, 1962, and J. S. Begando to Lyle Lanier, July 30, 1962, both in box 3, Administrative and Personnel Actions File.

4. Correspondence and memos, folder 2, July 1962–April 1963, Andrew Ivy Biographical and Correspondence Collection, Roosevelt University Archives, Chicago; "Ivy Becomes Professor at Roosevelt U.," *Chicago Tribune*, October 11, 1962, C15.

5. Ivy Cancer Research Foundation flyer, c. 1964, box 295, folder 7, Gloria Swanson Papers, Harry Ransom Center, University of Texas at Austin [hereafter,

Swanson Papers]; A. C. Ivy to Joseph S. Begando, February 12, 1963, box 3, Administrative and Personnel Actions File. See also "Auditorium Building," *Chicago Architecture Center*, https://www.architecture.org/learn/resources /buildings-of-chicago/building/auditorium-building/.

6. Lynn Weiner, "Who You Gonna Call? The Haunting of the Auditorium Theatre," *Roosevelt Review*, February 8, 2017, https://blogs.roosevelt .edu/review-archive/2017/02/08/who-you-gonna-call-the-haunting-of-the -auditorium-theatre/.

7. Abraham Ribicoff to Julius H. Miner, April 17, 1961, John F. Kennedy Presidential Library and Museum Archives, Boston, MA, https://www.jfklibrary .org/asset-viewer/archives/JFKWHSFLCW/006/JFKWHSFLCW-006 -009?image_identifier=JFKWHSFLCW-006-009-p0054.

8. Ribicoff to Miner; Elinor Langer, "Krebiozen: Nearly a Decade of Controversy Spent in Pursuit of 'Fair,' Government-Sponsored Test," *Science* 140, no. 3574 (June 28, 1963): 1383–85; Oveta Culp Hobby to Andrew Ivy and Stevan Durovic, May 25, 1954, box 3609, Records of the FDA, National Archives and Records Administration, College Park, MD [hereafter, FDA Records].

9. Ralph G. Smith to Stevan Durovic, June 9, 1961, box 8, folder 8, A. C. Ivy Papers, American Heritage Center, University of Wyoming, Laramie [hereafter, Ivy Papers].

10. National Cancer Institute, statement, September 29, 1961, US Department of Health, Education, and Welfare, Bethesda, Maryland, John F. Kennedy Presidential Library and Museum Archives, Boston, MA, https://www .jfklibrary.org/asset-viewer/archives/JFKWHSFLCW/006/JFKWHSFLCW -006-010?image_identifier=JFKWHSFLCW-006-010-p0035; A. C. Ivy, Stevan Durovic, and John Pick to Kenneth M. Endicott, July 17, 1962, in *Congressional Record* 108, part 11, July 20, 1962, 14287–91.

11. H. B. Andervont to A. C. Ivy, December 1, 1961, box 9, folder 13, Ivy Papers; Kenneth M. Endicott to A. C. Ivy and Stevan Durovic, March 7, 1962, box 441, folder 2, American Medical Association Historical Health Fraud and Alternative Medicine Collection, Chicago, IL [hereafter, AMA Collection].

12. Langer, "Krebiozen: Nearly a Decade of Controversy," 1385; Paul Douglas, statement, *Congressional Record* 108, part 11, July 20, 1962, 14287; A. C. Ivy, Stevan Durovic, and John Pick to Kenneth Endicott, 14291.

13. Ivy, Durovic, and Pick to Endicott, 14291.

14. A. C. Ivy to Paul Douglas, September 10, 1962, and Stevan Durovic, "Analysis of the Present Situation regarding Krebiozen," c. September 1962, both in box 307, Paul Douglas Papers, Abakanowicz Research Center, Chicago History Museum, Chicago, IL.

15. Walter Modell quoted in Philip J. Hilts, *Protecting America's Health: The FDA, Business, and One Hundred Years of Regulation* (New York: Alfred A. Knopf, 2003), 139.

16. Morton Mintz, "'Heroine' of FDA Keeps Bad Drug Off of Market," *Washington Post*, July 15, 1962, A1, A8; Jennifer Vanderbes, *Wonder Drug: The Secret*

History of Thalidomide in America and Its Hidden Victims (New York: Random House, 2023); Hilts, *Protecting America's Health*, 164–65.

17. "Federal Probe Launched into Drug Krebiozen," *Chicago Tribune*, January 16, 1963, 1, 10.

18. "Judge Miner Dies; Funeral Tomorrow," *Chicago Tribune*, March 14, 1963, 3.

19. Stevan Durovic and A. C. Ivy to Boisfeuillet Jones, January 24, 1963, box 3609, FDA Records. See also Elinor Langer, "Krebiozen: FDA Deadline Brings New, but Not the Final, Episode in Controversy over Cancer Drug," *Science* 141, no. 3575 (July 5, 1963): 31–33.

20. Drew Pearson, "Dad's Philosophy Guided Cooper," *Washington Post*, May 25, 1963, D13; Jack Mabley, "Fraud or Blessing—Krebiozen Controversy Must Be Resolved," *Chicago's American*, July 23, 1963, box S06, folder 12, AMA Collection; George Frazier, "A Certain Sadness," *Boston Herald*, June 7, 1963, box 441, folder 6, AMA Collection.

21. See, for example, Barbara Yuncker, "Krebiozen vs. Cancer—Proposal for a Final Test," *New York Post Daily Magazine*, September 30, 1960, 21.

22. "Catherine A. Manning," *Chicago Tribune*, January 16, 1992, sec. 2, 9; Donna Cornachio, "At 93, Author Finds It's Never Too Late for an Upside-Down Book," *New York Times*, July 9, 2000, WC14; Gloria Swanson to Julia A. E. Martens, August 22, 1963, and Gloria Swanson to President John F. Kennedy, March 5, 1963, both in box 299, folder 1, Swanson Papers.

23. Kenneth Endicott quoted in Siddhartha Mukherjee, *The Emperor of All Maladies: A Biography of Cancer* (New York: Scribner, 2011), 177; William D. Morain, "Krebiozen: Nineteen Years of Controversy," talk presented at Harvard University, March 18, 1968, box 446, folder 2, AMA Collection.

24. "Cecile Hoffman's IACVF and the Breakaway That Became the Cancer Control Society," *Cancer Control Society—Sonoma County Chapter*, November 26, 2011, https://cancercontrolsupport.blogspot.com/2011/11/. See also Mukherjee, *Emperor of All Maladies*, 60–72, 193–201.

25. Linda Lear, *Rachel Carson: Witness for Nature* (New York: Henry Holt, 1997), 365–68; Ellen Leopold, *A Darker Ribbon: Breast Cancer, Women, and Their Doctors in the Twentieth Century* (Boston: Beacon, 1999), 122–23.

26. Leopold, *Darker Ribbon*, 126–40; George Crile Jr., *Cancer and Common Sense* (New York: Viking, 1955), 102. See also Wolfgang Saxon, "Dr. George Crile Jr., Foe of Unneeded Surgery, Dies," *New York Times*, September 12, 1992, sec. 1, 10; Linda Lear, introduction to Rachel Carson, *Silent Spring* (Boston: Mariner, 2002), e-book.

27. Rachel Carson to Dorothy Freeman, March 19, 1963, in Martha Freeman, ed., *The Letters of Rachel Carson and Dorothy Freeman, 1952–1964* (Boston: Beacon, 1995), 442; Leopold, *Darker Ribbon*, 143–46.

28. Allan Morrison, "Hold Last Rites for Fashion, Food Expert Freda DeKnight," *Jet*, February 14, 1963, 40–41; William Barrow, "Tribute to a Lady Titan," *Negro Digest*, August 1963, 30–34; Donna Battle Pierce, "Freda

DeKnight: A 'Hidden Figure' and Titan of African-American Cuisine," February 16, 2017, NPR.org, https://www.npr.org/sections/thesalt/2017/02/16/514360992/meet-freda-deknight-a-hidden-figure-and-titan-of-african-american-food.

29. Nolene Hodges, "Girl with Cancer Waits Prayerfully; Puts Faith in Non-conforming Doctor," *News-Gazette* (Champaign, IL), June 16, 1963, Champaign County Historical Archives, Urbana Free Library, Urbana, IL; "Doctor Asks U.S. Ban Use of Krebiozen," *Decatur Herald* (IL), March 19, 1963, 19; "Diane Lindstrom Eagerly Uses Krebiozen and Delays Amputation of Her Leg," *Bedford Daily-Times* (IN), March 22, 1963, 9; Gene Cunningham, "Letters Pour in to Cancer Victim," *Rockford Register-Republic*, April 5, 1963, box 441, folder 3, AMA Collection.

30. "Laine Friedman Robins," June 17, 2003, Oregonlive.com, https://obits.oregonlive.com/us/obituaries/oregon/name/laine-robins-obituary?id=14103782; Robert P. Goldman, "The Fantastic Krebiozen Story," *Saturday Evening Post*, January 4, 1964, 18.

31. "March for Cancer Drug Vain, Wife to Fight On," *Daily News* (New York, NY), May 17, 1963, B3; Pearson, "Dad's Philosophy," D13.

32. William Moore, "Cancer Drug's Use Described for Congress," *Chicago Tribune*, May 15, 1963, C6; Tom Kelly, "Cancer Patients Beg for Drug," *Washington Daily News*, May 15, 1963, box 10, folder 6, Ivy Papers; "March for Cancer Drug"; "Report on the Krebiozen Delegation to Washington," c. June 1963, box 299, folder 1, Swanson Papers.

33. "Demonstrator Arrested at White House," *Washington Post*, June 5, 1963, B6; Percy Wood, "Ivy, Durovic Agree to Edict on Krebiozen," *Chicago Tribune*, June 7, 1963, A3.

34. "Durovic Cancels U.S. Test for Krebiozen," *Chicago Tribune*, July 13, 1963, 2; Percy Wood, "Ivy Pledges State Supply of Krebiozen," *Chicago Tribune*, July 16, 1963, A5; "Cancer Drug Supporters Picket White House," *Los Angeles Times*, August 7, 1963, 3, 21.

35. Goldman, "Fantastic Krebiozen Story," 18–19; "Food Editor Freda DeKnight Dies of Cancer after Courageous Fight," *Chicago Defender*, January 31, 1963, 1; Barrow, "Tribute to a Lady Titan," 34.

36. Stanley Buckles, "Cancer Victim Quits Krebiozen, Switches Doctors," *Rockford Morning Star* (IL), May 8, 1963, 1A-2A; Hodges, "Girl with Cancer Waits"; "Rockford Girl Is Not Helped by Treatments," *Daily Chronicle* (DeKalb, IL), August 7, 1963, 2; "Girl Shifts Treatment for Cancer," *Anderson Herald* (IN), September 19, 1963, 26; "Krebiozen Patient Dies of Bone Cancer," *Decatur Herald* (IL), October 30, 1963, 7.

37. Rachel Carson to Dorothy Freeman, May 2, 1963, in Freeman, ed., *Letters of Rachel Carson*, 457; Leopold, *Darker Ribbon*, 146–47; transcript of *American Experience: Rachel Carson*, May 28, 2019, https://www.pbs.org/wgbh/americanexperience/films/rachel-carson/#transcript.

38. Durovic and Ivy to Jones, January 24, 1963, box 3609, FDA Records; Boisfeuillet Jones to Stevan Durovic and A. C. Ivy, January 31, 1963, and Department

of Health, Education, and Welfare, "Report on the Current Status of Krebiozen," c. February 1963, both in box 441, folder 3, AMA Collection.

39. William F. Woo, "Long, Fruitless Efforts to Test Krebiozen," *St. Louis Post-Dispatch*, February 8, 1966, 3D; William F. Woo, "Wrangles Marked Krebiozen Inquiry," *St. Louis Post-Dispatch*, February 9, 1966, 3F. See also Joe Schwarcz, *Quack Quack: The Threat of Pseudoscience* (Toronto, ON: ECW, 2022), 28–32.

40. Matthew Hongoltz-Hetling, *If It Sounds like a Quack . . . : A Journey to the Fringes of American Medicine* (New York: Public Affairs, 2023), e-book, chap. 7.

41. Woo, "Wrangles Marked Krebiozen Inquiry"; Clifford B. Shane, interview by Fred L. Lofsvold and Robert G. Porter, April 23, 1980, in *History of the U.S. Food and Drug Administration*, 41–56, https://www.fda.gov/media/81130/download; "Chronology on Krebiozen," c. July 1963, box 3609, FDA Records.

42. National Cancer Institute, "Report of the Review Committee: Evaluation of Krebiozen Clinical Records," c. October 1963, box 9, folder 12, Ivy Papers; Shane interview; Elinor Langer, "Krebiozen: Government Indicts Sponsors of Alleged Cancer Drug; Ivy, Durovic among Those Named," *Science* 146, no. 3649 (December 4, 1964): 1282; Frances O. Kelsey to husband of Krebiozen patient, April 25, 1963, and Franklin Clark to Gertrude Gates, July 12, 1963, both in box 3609, FDA Records.

43. FDA, Promak Laboratories Inspection Report, May 8, 9, and 20, 1963, box 3609, FDA Records; Woo, "Wrangles Marked Krebiozen Inquiry." See also "A Brief History of the Pet Food Industry Part Two, The Introduction of Canned Pet Food Ken-L-Ration," *Epoch.pet*, March 19, 2019, https://epoch.pet/2019/03/19/a-brief-history-of-the-pet-food-industry-part-two-the-introduction-of-canned-pet-food-ken-l-ration/.

44. Woo, "Wrangles Marked Krebiozen Inquiry."

45. Woo, "Wrangles Marked Krebiozen Inquiry"; FDA, Promak Laboratories Inspection Report, May 8, 9, and 20, 1963.

46. FDA, Promak Laboratories Inspection Reports, June 5 and 8, 1963, box 3609, FDA Records; William F. Woo, "U.S. vs. Krebiozen—Fraud or Boon?," *St. Louis Post-Dispatch*, February 10, 1966, 3D.

47. Robert N. Palmer and Roland D. Sherman memorandum on visit to 100 S. Desplaines Street, Chicago, IL, June 19, 1963, and Robert N. Palmer memorandum on telephone call with James L. Griffin, June 10, 1963, both in box 3609, FDA Records; Percy Wood, "Durovic Sues Celebreeze in Krebiozen Row," *Chicago Tribune*, June 27, 1963, C5; "Judge Denies Injunction in Drug Inquiry," *Chicago Tribune*, July 4, 1963, C7; "Durovic Suit on Krebiozen Is Dismissed," *Chicago Tribune*, February 21, 1964, A5; Woo, "U.S. vs. Krebiozen," 3D; Stevan Durovic to Anthony J. Celebreeze, July 12, 1963, and Boisfeuillet Jones to Stevan Durovic, July 17, 1963, both in box 441, folder 5, AMA Collection.

48. Woo, "U.S. vs. Krebiozen," 3D; FDA, Promak Laboratories Inspection Report, June 8, 1963, box 3609, FDA Records; Robert N. Palmer affidavit,

August 2, 1963 (document supplied by FDA via Freedom of Information Act [FOIA] request). A couple of years later, during the fraud trial of Krebiozen's promoters, the government said that the drug's production cost was twenty-two cents an ampule (Sheila Wolfe, "U.S. Says $9.50 Is Charged for 22¢ Krebiozen," *Chicago Tribune*, October 2, 1965, A6).

49. Woo, "Long, Fruitless Efforts," 3D; Ronald Koziol, "Woman Fears Death, Steals Cancer Drug," *Chicago Tribune*, September 2, 1963, 3; Shane interview, 43; Raymond M. Mlecko, interview by Robert A. Tucker, June 15, 2003, 18–19, *History of the U.S. Food and Drug Administration*, https://www.fda.gov/media/81200/download.

50. "Creatine—Not Krebiozen!" *Medical World News*, September 27, 1963, 46–49; "Woman Chemist Directs Krebiozen Analysis," *Science News Letter*, September 28, 1963, 196; FDA, "Alma LeVant Hayden's Contributions to Regulatory Science," FDA History Exhibits, last revised January 20, 2022, https://www.fda.gov/about-fda/fda-history-exhibits/alma-levant-haydens-contributions-regulatory-science; Olivia Campbell, "The Chemist Who Exposed a Cancer Cure Fraud," *Beyond Curie*, April 1, 2022, https://oliviacampbell.substack.com/p/the-chemist-who-exposed-a-cancer.

51. "Creatine—Not Krebiozen," 46–49; Campbell, "Chemist Who Exposed"; FDA, "Alma LeVant Hayden's Contributions."

52. "Creatine—Not Krebiozen," 46–49; Robert C. Toth, "Krebiozen Found a Common Acid," *New York Times*, September 7, 1963, 21, 47; Daniel Banes, interview by James Harvey Young and Robert G. Porter, June 17, 1980, 30–42, in *History of the U.S. Food and Drug Administration*, https://www.fda.gov/media/81185/download; Warren R. Young, "What Ever Happened to Dr. Ivy?," *Life*, October 9, 1964, 110–12. See also John F. Allen, "Death Hastened by Cancer 'Cure' Pill, Probe Told; 2nd Drug Also Attacked," *San Francisco Examiner*, May 9, 1958, 15.

53. "Creatine—Not Krebiozen," 47; Stuart H. Loory, "'Fingerprints' End Hamburger Drug," *New York Herald-Tribune*, September 8, 1963, 1, 17.

54. Arthur J. Snider, "Krebiozen Foe Vindicated?," *Decatur Daily Review* (IL), September 16, 1963, 4.

55. National Cancer Institute, "Report of the Review Committee"; Elinor Langer, "Krebiozen: FDA, NIH Still on Trail of Anticancer Drug; and Congress on Trail of Agencies," *Science* 141, no. 3585 (September 13, 1963): 1021–23.

56. National Cancer Institute, "Report of the Review Committee."

57. Kenneth Endicott, "Clinical Trial of 'Krebiozen' under National Cancer Institute Sponsorship," October 15, 1963, box 9, folder 13, Ivy Papers.

58. "FDA Moves to Prosecute Sponsors of Drug," *Medical World News*, September 27, 1963, 49.

59. Yuncker, "Krebiozen vs. Cancer—Proposal for a Final Test," 21; Vanderbes, *Wonder Drug*. See also James Harvey Young and Richard E. McFayden, "The Koch Cancer Treatment," *Journal of the History of Medicine and Allied Sciences* 53, no. 3 (July 1998): 254–84.

Chapter 6. The Emperor's New Clothes

1. "The Making of a Maverick," *Time*, January 16, 1950, http://content.time .com/time/magazine/article/0,9171,811716,00.html; "Paul Douglas Dies," *Chicago Tribune*, September 25, 1976, sec. 1, 1, 5.

2. Roger Biles, *Crusading Liberal: Paul H. Douglas of Illinois* (DeKalb: Northern Illinois University Press, 2002), 129; Paul H. Douglas, *In the Fullness of Time* (New York: Harcourt Brace Jovanovich, 1972), 336–45, 390–99.

3. Biles, *Crusading Liberal*, 212.

4. "FDA Tags Krebiozen as Common Amino Acid," *Chicago Tribune*, September 7, 1963, N1, N4; Stevan Durovic to Anthony J. Celebreeze, September 11, 1963, box 9, folder 13, A. C. Ivy Papers, American Heritage Center, University of Wyoming, Laramie [hereafter, Ivy Papers]; Earl Ubell, "Krebiozen Champions— a Fight for Life," *New York Herald-Tribune*, September 13, 1963, series 002/01/01, box 1, folder 10, George Stoddard Papers, University of Illinois-Chicago Archives; "Krebiozen and Cancer: Thirteen Years of Bitter Conflict," *YouTube*, posted by William Kronick, https://www.youtube.com/watch?v=0TGjm7wIyUk.

5. Boisfeuillet Jones to Stevan Durovic, September 26, 1963, box 9, folder 13, Ivy Papers; Arthur J. Snider, "Sad Valedictory to Dr. Ivy; the Reporters Walked Out," *Chicago Daily News*, c. October 1963, series 002/01/01, box 1, folder 8, George Stoddard Papers, University of Illinois-Chicago Archives; George Frazier to Howard Shuman, December 23, 1963, box 309, Paul Douglas Papers, Abakanowicz Research Center, Chicago History Museum [hereafter, Douglas Papers].

6. Howard E. Shuman, interview by Donald A. Ritchie, Oral History Project, United States Senate Historical Office, August 19, 1987, 425–26, https://www .senate.gov/about/resources/pdf/shuman-howard-e-full-transcript-with-index .pdf; Howard E. Shuman, "Memo for Krebiozen Files," July 29, 1988, series 26/20/74, box 7, Howard E. Shuman Papers, University of Illinois at Urbana-Champaign Archives [hereafter, Shuman Papers]; Miles H. Robinson and Howard E. Shuman, "Qualifications of Committee Preparing Report," December 4, 1963, box 1282, Douglas Papers; Thomas T. Fenton, "Physician Asks 'Fair Deal' for Controversial Krebiozen," *Baltimore Sun*, January 3, 1964, 19, 34. See also "Unproven Methods of Cancer Treatment: National Health Federation," *CA* 41, no. 1 (January/February 1991): 61–64.

7. Paul H. Douglas, "FDA Mistaken, Krebiozen Not Creatine: NCI Judgment of Cases Biased and Irrelevant: Evidence Justifies Fair Test Now," reprint from *Congressional Record*, December 6, 1963, box 7, Shuman Papers; Barbara Widmar, "Sen. Douglas' Krebiozen Report Attacks FDA on 5 Counts," *Champaign-Urbana Courier* (IL), December 12, 1963, 24; Barbara Widmar, "Report to Douglas Calls FDA Color Blind," *Champaign-Urbana Courier*, December 15, 1963, 22, 24.

8. Paul H. Douglas to Lyndon B. Johnson, January 31, 1964, box 309, Douglas Papers (emphasis in original); Howard Shuman, "Memorandum for the File," June 9, 1964, box 7, Shuman Papers.

9. Shuman, "Memorandum." See also Douglas, *In the Fullness of Time*, 233–35; Shuman interview.

10. Donald F. Hornig to Paul H. Douglas, April 6, 1964, and Paul H. Douglas to Donald F. Hornig, April 10, 1964, both in box 1281, Douglas Papers. See also Shuman, "Memorandum."

11. Douglas, "FDA Mistaken"; Raymond M. Rice to Paul Douglas, December 19, 1963, box 1278, Douglas Papers.

12. George D. Stoddard, *"Krebiozen": The Great Cancer Mystery* (Boston: Beacon, 1955), 37.

13. "Krebiozen Story: Secrecy Brought Drug Curb," *Denver Post*, January 9, 1964, in *Congressional Record* 110, part 2, February 7, 1964, 2428.

14. Shuman, "Memorandum."

15. Paul H. Douglas to Andrew C. Ivy and Stevan Durovic, April 21, 1964, box 1283, Douglas Papers; Shuman, "Memorandum."

16. "Telephone Conversation between Howard Shuman and Dr. Stevan Durovic on May 8, 1964," box 1283, Douglas Papers; Shuman, "Memorandum."

17. Shuman, "Memorandum."

18. Shuman, "Memorandum."

19. Paul H. Douglas to Andrew C. Ivy and Stevan Durovic, June 11, 1964, Stevan Durovic to Paul H. Douglas, May 31, 1964, and Howard E. Shuman to Paul Douglas, November 4, 1964, all in box 1283, Douglas Papers.

20. Roy Gibbons, "Postpone Ban on Krebiozen Distribution," *Chicago Tribune*, January 11, 1964, 5; Jack Levine, "1500 Want FDA Investigated on Krebiozen," *Kings County Chronicle* (NY), February 11, 1964, 12; Herbert Bailey to Andrew C. Ivy, October 31, 1963, box 1283, Douglas Papers.

21. Bailey to Ivy, October 31, 1963; Edward T. Carmody to Charles M. Byrnes, March 5, 1964, box 87, folder 17, Ivy Papers.

22. "Krebiozen: What the Fighting Is All About," *Chicago Tribune*, May 30, 1964, D6.

23. "Krebiozen and Cancer"; "Krebiozen Film Will Be Shown," *Long Branch Daily Record* (NJ), November 26, 1965, 3.

24. Cathy Hodnett to Lyndon B. Johnson, February 2, 1965, and "Krebiozen Fact Sheet—Mrs. Julie Hodnett and Her Daughter Cathy," February 25, 1966, both in series HE 4, box 15, Lyndon Baines Johnson Papers, Lyndon Baines Johnson Library, Austin, TX, White House Central Files; Sandra Otto Cummings, "Controversy Rages and So Does Cancer," *Asbury Park Press* (NJ), April 15, 1962, 1, 4; Cathy Hodnett flyer, box 296, folder 5, Gloria Swanson Papers, Harry Ransom Center, University of Texas at Austin. Cathy Hodnett died of cancer in 1967; see "Krebiozen Poster Girl of '63 Dies," *Asbury Park Press* (NJ), February 12, 1967, 1.

25. Gertrude Brou to Lyndon B. Johnson, c. May 1964, box 3770, Records of the Food and Drug Administration, National Archives and Records Administration, College Park, MD; "Rules against Krebiozen for Jailed Woman," *Chicago Tribune*, July 23, 1964, 8; Nancy Taylor, "Mrs. Brou—a 96-Pound Fighter," *Hollywood Sun-Tattler* (FL), July 30, 1964, 1A, 3A; Simon Bloom, "Krebiozen

Cancer Patients Fight Back," *American Jewish Ledger* (Newark, NJ), February 27, 1965, box 442, folder 3, American Medical Association Historical Health Fraud and Alternative Medicine Collection, Chicago, IL.

26. "Quackery and Tragedy Are Twins," *Chicago Daily News*, October 30, 1963, 10; "Political Pressure vs. Medical Decisions," *Consumer Reports*, February 1964, 95; Howard Margolis, "The Curious Case of Krebiozen," *Bulletin of Atomic Scientists*, March 1964, 29.

27. Warren R. Young, "What Ever Happened to Dr. Ivy?," *Life*, October 9, 1964, 110–26; A. C. Ivy to *Life* magazine, October 19, 1964, AMA Collection, box 442, folder 2, American Medical Association Historical Health Fraud and Alternative Medicine Collection, Chicago, IL.

28. "Act to Indict in Probe of Krebiozen," *Chicago Tribune*, October 28, 1964, 1; Percy Wood, "Indict Dr. Ivy on Krebiozen," *Chicago Tribune*, November 18, 1964, 1, 4; George Murray, "Dr. Durovic Story: $1.7 Million Sent 'to Repay Loans,'" *Chicago's American*, October 30, 1964, 1, 3; Sheila Wolfe, "U.S. Says $9.50 Is Charged for 22¢ Krebiozen," *Chicago Tribune*, October 2, 1965, A6.

29. "Demonstrators Eye Anti-Cancer Drug," *Fort Lauderdale News*, October 31, 1964, 11; Percy Wood, "'Not Guilty,' Says Dr. Ivy; Trial Jan. 11," *Chicago Tribune*, November 19, 1964, 11; "Ivy Loses on Krebiozen Release," *Chicago Tribune*, December 12, 1964, 3.

30. Wood, "Not Guilty," 11; David Smothers, "Awaits Trial Coming Month," *DeKalb Chronicle* (IL), December 3, 1964, folder 3, Andrew Ivy Biographical and Correspondence Collection, Roosevelt University Archives, Chicago, IL [hereafter, Ivy Roosevelt Collection].

31. "Judge Denies Injunction in Drug Inquiry," *Chicago Tribune*, July 4, 1963, C7; Edward Baumann and Jack Houston, "Julius Hoffman, Judge at Trial of 'Chicago 7,'" *Chicago Tribune*, June 2, 1983, sec. 1, 12; Joseph C. Goulden, *The Benchwarmers: The Private World of the Powerful Federal Judges* (New York: Weybright and Talley, 1974), 137–42. See also Douglas O. Linder, "'The Chicago Eight' (or 'Chicago Seven') Trial (1969–1970)," *Famous Trials*, n.d., https://famous-trials.com/chicago8.

32. "Judge Irked by Defense, Defers Krebiozen Trial," *Chicago Tribune*, December 22, 1964, 1; John O'Brien, "Trial of Krebiozen Case Set for April 5," *Chicago Tribune*, January 16, 1965, 6; "Dismissals in Krebiozen Case Denied," *Stevens Point Daily Journal* (WI), January 15, 1965, 13; "Krebiozen Case Figure Causes Furor by Absence," *Tulsa Daily World*, January 16, 1965, 7; A. C. Ivy to Miles H. Robinson, January 19, 1965, box 86, folder 7, Ivy Papers.

33. "Ivy Loses Bid for Own Trial on Krebiozen," *Chicago Tribune*, April 3, 1965, A3; Sheila Wolfe, "Trial of Dr. Ivy, Durovics in Krebiozen Case Opens," *Chicago Tribune*, April 29, 1965, N1, N8; Sheila Wolfe, "Jury Sworn in to Try Dr. Ivy and Durovics," *Chicago Tribune*, May 1, 1965, 16.

34. Horton Trautman, "U.S. Charges 4 with Lies on Krebiozen," *Chicago Daily News*, May 3, 1965, 1, 44; Horton Trautman, "Krebiozen Defense Charges Conspiracy," *Chicago Daily News*, May 4, 1965, 11.

35. Wood, "Indict Dr. Ivy," 4; Sheila Wolfe, "U.S. Rests Its Case in Trial on Krebiozen," *Chicago Tribune*, October 6, 1965, E11; "Mineral Oil Purchases by Durovic Told," *Chicago Tribune*, June 8, 1965, 19; William F. Woo, "The Long Battle over Krebiozen," *St. Louis Post-Dispatch*, February 6, 1966, 1G, 8G; "Durovic Ill; His Krebiozen Trial Delayed," *Chicago Tribune*, June 15, 1965, C13; Sheila Wolfe, "Judge Orders Ailing Durovic to Courtroom," June 17, 1965, D7; Sheila Wolfe, "Jury Excused in Krebiozen Trial Delay," *Chicago Tribune*, August 3, 1965, A7.

36. Sheila Wolfe, "Trial Is Told Ivy OK'd Pleas for Krebiozen," *Chicago Tribune*, May 6, 1965, 18; Sheila Wolfe, "U.S. Thwarted in Krebiozen Probe: Agent," *Chicago Tribune*, May 15, 1965, N9; Sheila Wolfe, "Thalidomide Prober Called in Ivy's Trial," *Chicago Tribune*, June 24, 1965, D27; Sheila Wolfe, "Doctor Tells Testing Cost of Krebiozen," *Chicago Tribune*, July 22, 1965, D16; Sheila Wolfe, "U.S. Aid Tells of Oil Content in Krebiozen," *Chicago Tribune*, September 2, 1965, A7.

37. "Pleas Denied for Acquittal on Krebiozen," *Chicago Tribune*, October 9, 1965, N8; Woo, "Long Battle," 1G; Sheila Wolfe, "Medic Credits Cancer Cure to Krebiozen," *Chicago Tribune*, October 29, 1965, 7; "Disputes Claim Krebiozen Is Only Creatine," *Chicago Tribune*, October 16, 1965, 7; Scott Anderson, "Rough Draft of Talk Given in Fayetteville, Arkansas," April 20, 1974, box 9, Shuman Papers; "Judge Defends Jury System, Lashes at Ivy," *Chicago Tribune*, April 1, 1965, F7.

38. Letter to Andrew Ivy, October 16, 1963, folder 2, Ivy Roosevelt Collection; Sheila Wolfe, "Federal Agent Tells How He Got Krebiozen," *Chicago Tribune*, June 19, 1965, A9; Sheila Wolfe, "Offers Bank Data in Cancer Drug Trial," *Chicago Tribune*, July 15, 1965, A3; Woo, "Long Battle," 1G.

39. Sheila Wolfe, "Dr. Ivy Takes Stand in 8th Month of Trial," *Chicago Tribune*, December 2, 1965, D1; Sheila Wolfe, "Dr. Ivy Tells of U.S. Plan to Test Drug," *Chicago Tribune*, December 3, 1965, A8; M. W. Newman, "Andrew Ivy, Man on Trial," *Chicago Daily News*, December 3, 1965, 54; Sheila Wolfe, "Cancer Jurors Shown Powders," *Chicago Tribune*, December 4, 1965, 5; Sheila Wolfe, "Ivy Says Test of Krebiozen Was Promised," *Chicago Tribune*, December 7, 1965, B17; Max Sonderby, "Cartload of Honors, Testimonials Presented in Dr. Ivy's Defense," *Chicago Sun-Times*, December 8, 1965, folder 4, Ivy Roosevelt Collection.

40. Horton Trautman, "Dr. Ivy Admits Scant Experience," *Chicago Daily News*, December 8, 1965, folder 4, Ivy Roosevelt Collection; Sheila Wolfe, "Dr. Ivy Tells of Tumor Growth in Spite of Krebiozen," *Chicago Tribune*, December 15, 1965, D2; Sheila Wolfe, "Made Nothing on Krebiozen, Dr. Ivy Says," *Chicago Tribune*, December 18, 1965, 10; Sheila Wolfe, "Defense Rests in Krebiozen Fraud Trial," *Chicago Tribune*, December 22, 1965, A8; Sheila Wolfe, "U.S. Ends Case in Krebiozen Fraud Trial," *Chicago Tribune*, December 31, 1965, 8.

41. D. Arthur Connelly closing argument, January 12, 1966, box 81, folder 2, Ivy Papers; Horton Trautman, "U.S. Reads a Fairy Tale to Sum Up Krebiozen Case," *Chicago Daily News*, January 12, 1966, 1, 11; Sheila Wolfe, "Krebiozen Is

a Fairy Tale, Jurors Told," *Chicago Tribune*, January 13, 1966, B10; Sheila Wolfe, "U.S. Questions Ivy's Motives on Krebiozen," *Chicago Tribune*, January 14, 1966, A5.

42. Horton Trautman, "Krebiozen Jury Hears Dr. Ivy," *Chicago Daily News*, December 1, 1965, 1, 10; Horton Trautman, "Krebiozen Jury Gets Final Pleas," *Chicago Daily News*, January 13, 1966, 3; Horton Trautman, "Dr. Ivy's Lawyer Turns to Poetry," *Chicago Daily News*, January 18, 1966, 5; Sheila Wolfe, "Ivy's 'Quest for Test' of Krebiozen Called Frustrating," *Chicago Tribune*, January 18, 1966, A2; Horton Trautman, "Help Cancer Cure Hopes, Jury Asked," *Chicago Daily News*, January 21, 1966, 3.

43. Shelia Wolfe, "Krebiozen Trial Nears Jury," *Chicago Tribune*, January 25, 1966, 1–2; "Jury Ponders Krebiozen Case Verdict," *Chicago Tribune*, January 27, 1966, sec. 3, 12; Woo, "Long Battle," 1G.

44. Sheila Wolfe, "Jury Releases 3 in Krebiozen Case; Debates on Dr. Durovic," *Chicago Tribune*, January 30, 1966, 1–2; "Krebiozen Jurors Free 3," *Chicago Sun-Times*, January 30, 1966, 1, 22.

45. Sheila Wolfe, "Krebiozen Trial Juror Collapses," *Chicago Tribune*, January 31, 1966, 1–2; Horton Trautman, "Dr. Durovic Innocent," *Chicago Daily News*, January 31, 1966, 1, 8; Norman Glubok, "Jurors Tell Why," *Chicago Daily News*, January 31, 1966, 1, 8; Sheila Wolfe, "Jury Clears Dr. Durovic of 40 Counts," *Chicago Tribune*, February 1, 1966, 1, 8; John O'Brien, "How Jury Reached Krebiozen Decision," *Chicago Tribune*, February 1, 1966, 9.

46. Clifford B. Shane, interview by Fred L. Lofsvold and Robert G. Porter, April 23, 1980, 47–50, *History of the U.S. Food and Drug Administration*, https://www.fda.gov/media/81130/download; Wolfe, "U.S. Says $9.50 Is Charged," A6; Robert H. Collins, "Woman Admits Sending Mail on Krebiozen to 12 Jurors," *St. Louis Post-Dispatch*, February 18, 1966, 1, 4; "Meat Cutters' Sign Slices World News into Meaty Slogans," *Chicago Tribune*, February 17, 1966, F6; Robert H. Collins, "Krebiozen Jury Inquiry Sought by U.S. Attorney," *St. Louis Post-Dispatch*, February 20, 1966, 1, 15; Julius J. Hoffman contempt certificate against Julius L. Sherwin, c. 1966, and Kitty Schumacher to Julius J. Hoffman, November 8, 1964, and July 16, 1965, all in Julius J. Hoffman Papers, Abakanowicz Research Center, Chicago History Museum, box 24. See also Hilton E. Hanna and Joseph Belsky, *Picket and the Pen: The Pat Gorman Story* (Yonkers, NY: American Institute of Social Science, 1960); Patricia Spain Ward, "'Who Will Bell the Cat?' Andrew C. Ivy and Krebiozen," *Bulletin of the History of Medicine* 58, no. 1 (Spring 1984): 49–52.

47. Robert H. Collins, "Three on Jury Call Foreman Pro-Krebiozen," *St. Louis Post-Dispatch*, February 27, 1966, 1, 24; Robert H. Collins, "Jurors Recall Effort to Ruin Krebiozen Case," *St. Louis Post-Dispatch*, February 28, 1966, 1, 11; Robert H. Collins, "Krebiozen Jury Figure Tells of His Role," *St. Louis Post-Dispatch*, March 30, 1966, 5A; Robert H. Collins, "Juror Admits Reading Story on Krebiozen," *St. Louis Post-Dispatch*, May 8, 1966, 1, 20; Robert H. Collins, "Plot to Acquit 4 Defendants in Krebiozen Trial Charged," *St. Louis Post-Dispatch*,

August 1, 1966, 3A; Robert H. Collins, "Krebiozen Articles Cited in Testimony," *St. Louis Post-Dispatch*, January 10, 1969, 4A.

48. Robert H. Collins, "Krebiozen Case Juror Found Guilty," *St. Louis Post-Dispatch*, January 16, 1969, 1, 10; Robert Enstad, "Clear Woman on Krebiozen Jury Letters," *Chicago Tribune*, March 28, 1968, sec. 2, 26.

49. John O'Brien, "Indict Durovic as Tax Cheat," *Chicago Tribune*, March 11, 1966, 1–2; Robert H. Collins, "Marko Durovic Charges U.S. Persecutes Him and Brother," *St. Louis Post-Dispatch*, March 21, 1966, 14A; "Durovics Sued for $11,787 in Drug Trial," *Chicago Tribune*, March 29, 1966, B9.

50. "Ivy Drops Stoddard Libel Suit," *Chicago Tribune*, June 11, 1966, 9.

51. Dorothy Wetzel, "New Krebiozen Suit Cites U.I.," *Champaign-Urbana Courier*, February 16, 1966, 3; Barry Schweid, "High Court Appeal Asked on Krebiozen," *Champaign-Urbana Courier*, November 22, 1967, 6; "Deny Hearing in Krebiozen's Case Appeal," *Chicago Tribune*, January 16, 1968, sec. 1, 4; "11 Senators Ask FDA Test on Krebiozen," *Chicago Tribune*, April 2, 1966, 12; "Krebiozen May Cause Cancer, U.S. Aid Says," *Chicago Tribune*, April 21, 1966, D9; "Statement by Commissioner Goddard," March 31, 1966, box 8, folder 8, Ivy Papers (emphasis in original).

52. Samuel Stafford, "'Don't Ever Get Cancer—It's No Joke,'" *Washington Daily News*, March 29, 1966, 5; "Stage Sit-In; Urge FDA Free Krebiozen," *Chicago Tribune*, March 29, 1966, 1; "FDA Ousts Backers of Krebiozen," *Akron Beacon Journal* (Ohio), March 29, 1966, A1-A2.

53. "Food and Drug Administration's Summary of Important Facts Developed during the Krebiozen Case," c. 1966, box 4405, Records of the Food and Drug Administration, National Archives and Records Administration, College Park, MD; "New Bill Spells End to Krebiozen," *Champaign-Urbana Courier*, October 12, 1973, 6; Ronald Kotulak, "New Law Bans Sale of Krebiozen in Illinois," *Chicago Tribune*, October 12, 1973, A14; "Court Backs Ban on Krebiozen," *Chicago Tribune*, October 16, 1973, 3.

Conclusion

1. "Dr. Ivy Names Anti-cancer Substance 'Carcalon,'" and "How and Why Dr. Ivy Coined Name 'Carcalon,'" *Ivy Cancer News*, June 1967, 1, 3–4, box 94, folder 11, A. C. Ivy Papers, American Heritage Center, University of Wyoming, Laramie. For more on George Crane and his promotion of Carcalon, see George W. Crane, "The Worry Clinic," *Dixon Evening Telegraph* (IL), September 14, 1971, 12; Robert McG. Thomas Jr., "George W. Crane Dies at 94; Advised with 'Horse Sense,'" *New York Times*, July 19, 1995, D20.

2. David Kleinerman to Andrew C. Ivy, June 8, 1967, and Thaddeus P. Kawalek to Robert J. Pitchell, December 7, 1964, both in folders 3–4, Andrew Ivy Biographical and Correspondence Collection, Roosevelt University Archives, Chicago, IL; "Lab Move Completed," *Ivy Cancer News*, December 1967, 4, "ICRF Executive Director Gives Annual Report," *Ivy Cancer News*, December 1968, 1–2,

and "Ivy Cancer Research Foundation Marks 10th Anniversary," *Ivy Cancer News*, September 1969, 1, 4, all in box 295, folder 8, Gloria Swanson Papers, Harry Ransom Center, University of Texas at Austin; Earl L. Meyers to W. C. Johnson, December 4, 1968, box 4405, Records of the Food and Drug Administration, National Archives and Records Administration, College Park, MD.

3. Daniel Banes interviewed by James Harvey Young and Robert G. Porter, June 17, 1980, 41–42, *History of the U.S. Food and Drug Administration*, https:// www.fda.gov/media/81185/download; D. B. Dill, "A. C. Ivy—Reminiscences," *Physiologist* 22, no. 5 (October 1979): 21; transcript of Andrew Ivy on *Target: News*, WBBM-TV, Chicago, November 22, 1964, box 8, folder 3, A. C. Ivy Papers, American Heritage Center, University of Wyoming; Barbara Yuncker, "Krebiozen vs. Cancer: The Sideshows," *New York Post Daily Magazine*, October 2, 1960, 5; Warren R. Young, "What Ever Happened to Dr. Ivy?," *Life*, October 9, 1964, 126.

4. Yuncker, "Krebiozen vs. Cancer," 5; Arthur J. Snider, "Dr. Ivy Standing Pat in Krebiozen Fight," *Chicago Daily News*, August 26, 1961, 3; Young, "What Ever Happened to Dr. Ivy?," 121–22; A. C. Ivy to Miles H. Robinson, December 13, 1965, box 1283, Paul Douglas Papers, Abakanowicz Research Center, Chicago History Museum.

5. Young, "What Ever Happened to Dr. Ivy?," 122; Fred W. Fitz to J. Roscoe Miller, July 20, 1949, box 79, folder 3, J. Roscoe Miller Papers, Northwestern University Archives, Evanston, IL.

6. Leonard Keene Hirshberg, "The Dead Mending the Living," *Pittsburgh Sun-Telegraph*, July 30, 1944, American Weekly, sec. 8; Enrico Fantoni, "Nuclear Island: The Secret Post–WWII Mega Lab Investigated," *Wired*, February 14, 2011, https://www.wired.co.uk/article/nuclear-island?page=all.

7. "Second Report by President Stoddard to Joint Legislative Committee," March 25, 1953, in George D. Stoddard, *"Krebiozen": The Great Cancer Mystery* (Boston: Beacon, 1955), 227.

8. William D. Morain, "Krebiozen: Nineteen Years of Controversy," talk presented at Harvard University, March 18, 1968, box 446, folder 2, American Medical Association Historical Health Fraud and Alternative Medicine Collection, Chicago, IL. See also "The Ticker and the Flicker," *Time*, January 2, 1950, https://content.time.com/time/subscriber/article/0,33009,780202,00.html.

9. Snider, "Dr. Ivy Standing Pat," 3.

10. Clark Kerr, *The Uses of the University*, 5th ed. (Cambridge, MA: Harvard University Press, 2001), 1–34.

11. Robert B. Throckmorton to F. J. L. Blasingame, September 17, 1963, box 441, folder 6, American Medical Association Historical Health Fraud and Alternative Medicine Collection, Chicago, IL.

12. Elinor Langer, "The Krebiozen Case: What Happened in Chicago," *Science* 151, no. 3714 (March 4, 1966): 1061–64.

13. James Harvey Young, *American Health Quackery: Collected Essays* (Princeton, NJ: Princeton University Press, 1992), 24–25; Eric S. Juhnke, *Quacks and Crusaders: The Fabulous Careers of John Brinkley, Norman Baker, and Harry Hoxsey*

(Lawrence: University Press of Kansas, 2002), 118. See also James C. Petersen and Gerald E. Markle, "Politics and Science in the Laetrile Controversy," *Social Studies of Science* 9 (1979): 139–66.

14. Juhnke, *Quacks and Crusaders*, 107.

15. "Libonati Will Seek to Curb Stoddard's Power at U.I.," *Champaign-Urbana Courier* (IL), December 19, 1952, series 2/10/20, box 28, George D. Stoddard Papers, University of Illinois at Urbana-Champaign Archives.

16. Laine Friedman to editor of *Saturday Evening Post*, January 11, 1964, box 1279, Paul Douglas Papers, Abakanowicz Research Center, Chicago History Museum; Barbara R. Lillis, "Krebiozen" (letter to the editor), *Saturday Evening Post*, February 1, 1964, 4; Ellen Leopold, *A Darker Ribbon: Breast Cancer, Women, and Their Doctors in the Twentieth Century* (Boston: Beacon, 1999), 137, 144; Bruno Klopfer, "Psychological Variables in Human Cancer," *Journal of Projective Techniques* 21, no. 4 (December 1957): 337–39; Harry Collins and Trevor Pinch, *Dr. Golem: How to Think about Medicine* (Chicago: University of Chicago Press, 2005), e-book, introduction.

17. Juhnke, *Quacks and Crusaders*; James Harvey Young and Richard E. McFayden, "The Koch Cancer Treatment," *Journal of the History of Medicine and Allied Sciences* 53, no. 3 (July 1998): 254–84.

18. Lee Edson, "Why Laetrile Won't Go Away," *New York Times Magazine*, November 27, 1977, 41; Charles G. Moertel, Thomas R. Fleming, Joseph Rubin, Larry K. Kvols, Gregory Sarna, Robert Koch, Violante E. Currie, Charles W. Young, Stephen E. Jones, and J. Paul Davignon, "A Clinical Trial of Amygdalin (Laetrile) in the Treatment of Human Cancer," *New England Journal of Medicine* 306, no. 4 (January 28, 1982): 201. See also Benjamin Wilson, "The Rise and Fall of Laetrile," May 18, 2019, *Quackwatch*, https://quackwatch.org/related/Cancer/laetrile/; Young, *American Health Quackery*, 205–55.

19. Candice Basterfield, Scott O. Lilienfeld, Shauna M. Bowes, and Thomas H. Costello, "The Nobel Disease: When Intelligence Fails to Protect against Irrationality," *Skeptical Inquirer* 44, no. 3 (May/June 2020), https://skepticalinquirer.org/2020/05/the-nobel-disease-when-intelligence-fails-to-protect-against-irrationality/. See also Paul A. Offit, *Do You Believe in Magic? The Sense and Nonsense of Alternative Medicine* (New York: Harper, 2013), e-book, chap. 2.

20. Offit, *Do You Believe in Magic?* chaps. 8–9.

21. John T. Flynn, "Krebiozen and Faith" (letter to the editor), *Science* 152, no. 3722 (April 29, 1966): 592.

22. "George Stoddard Dies at 84; Educator Led 4 Universities," *New York Times*, December 29, 1981, D17; George Stoddard, "Notes for a Krebiozen Novel," series 002/01/01, box 1, folder 3, George Stoddard Papers, University of Illinois-Chicago Archives.

23. Arthur J. Snider, "Krebiozen Foe Vindicated?," *Decatur Daily Review* (IL), September 16, 1963, 4; Paul H. Douglas, *In the Fullness of Time: The Memoirs of Paul H. Douglas* (New York: Harcourt Brace Jovanovich, 1972), 336–45; "Paul H. Douglas," *Chicago Tribune*, September 26, 1976, A4.

24. William L. Raby, "The Reluctant Taxpayer," *San Bernardino County Sun*, September 24, 1970, 15; "Seized on 312 Parking Tickets," *Chicago Tribune*, September 9, 1971, 3; Jack Star, "So You Scoff at Parking Tickets," *Chicago Tribune Magazine*, April 1, 1973, 29; "Services Set for Durovic, Figure in Krebiozen Case," *Chicago Tribune*, December 7, 1976, sec. 3, 14.

25. Robert H. Collins, "Dr. Durovic Now in Switzerland for Treatment of Tuberculosis," *St. Louis Post-Dispatch*, May 6, 1966, 3A. Stevan Durovic's death date is taken from information at ancestry.com.

26. Jack Mabley, "Doctor Still Certain of Vindication," *Chicago Tribune*, June 2, 1975, 4; Ronald Kotulak, "Dr. Ivy, Krebiozen's Tragic Figure, to Retire," *Chicago Tribune*, May 16, 1976, 40; "Dr. Andrew Ivy Rites Set; Backed Krebiozen," *Chicago Tribune*, February 9, 1978, 6.

27. Patricia Spain Ward, "100 Years," '*Scope* 8, no. 3 (1981–82): 25. See also Patricia Spain Ward, "'Who Will Bell the Cat?' Andrew C. Ivy and Krebiozen," *Bulletin of the History of Medicine* 58, no. 1 (Spring 1984): 28–52.

28. Clifford B. Shane, interview by Fred L. Lofsvold and Robert G. Porter, April 23, 1980, 53–54, *History of the U.S. Food and Drug Administration*, https://www.fda.gov/media/81130/download. The FDA never dropped fraud investigations entirely, and more recently it has sought to crack down on several instances of potential quackery (Matthew Hongoltz-Hetling, *If It Sounds like a Quack . . .: A Journey to the Fringes of American Medicine* [New York: Public Affairs, 2023]).

29. Andrew Conway Ivy, interviewed and recorded by James David Boyle, November 4, 1968 (transcript), 21, National Library of Medicine, https://oculus.nlm.nih.gov/cgi/t/text/text-idx?c=oralhist;cc=oralhist;rgn=main;view=text;idno=2935142r; Young, "What Ever Happened to Dr. Ivy?," 126.

30. F. Perry Wilson, *How Medicine Works and When It Doesn't: Learning Who to Trust to Get and Stay Healthy* (New York: Grand Central, 2023), e-book, chap. 3; George Crile Jr., *Cancer and Common Sense* (New York: Viking, 1955), 102.

Index

Independent Cancer Research Foundation, 96–98, 100, 103, 114, 188n31
Institute of Medicine of Chicago, 44, 61
International Association of Cancer Victims and Friends, 114
Iowa Child Welfare Research Station, 17, 24. *See also* University of Iowa
Ivy, Andrew, 1–2, 10–15, *22, 75, 130, 146*; and academic freedom, 67; and AMA, 22, 31, 50, 69, 155; ambition of, 154, 161–62; and American Cancer Society, 69, 102–4, 155; and American Physiological Society, 152; and animal welfare activists, 23; anti-discrimination pamphlet by, 22; and Herbert Bailey, 88–89, 91, 93, 99, 101, 157; and Joseph Begando, 108; and Franklin Bing, 47–48, 50, 76; and Randolph Bohrer, *75*, 81, 82; and John Boyle, 36, 71–73, 81–82, 99; cancer theories of, 11, 32–33, 34, 95, 154; and Carcalon, 151–52, 161; and Anton J. Carlson, 21, 47, 94, 152; and Chicago Medical Society, 48, 50–53, 155; childhood of, 68; clinical experience of, 35, 54, 143–44; and Warren Cole, 52, 57; and George Crane, 151; and Paul Douglas, 43, 70, 99, 130–36, 156; Stevan Durovic, defenses of, 36, 100, 112; Durovic, differences with, 35–36, 43–44, 99–100, 134, 135, 142; Durovic, first meetings with, 31–33, 154; and FDA 101–2, 109–10, 120–28, 130–31, 143, 151–52, 155; final years of, 15, 161–62; fundraising events for, 99, 100; fundraising prowess of, 23, 52, 65, 71–72, 154; and Coleman Griffith, 51, 64–65, 71–72; and HEW, 101–2, 113, 120, 123, 131; and Julius Hoffman, 140–41, 143, 144; and hope in medicine, 15, 67, 161–62; and Harry Hoxsey, 69; and Illinois legislature, 52, 65–67, 70–72, 89, 107, 155; journalism's

coverage of, 23, 74, 131, 138–39, 152–54, 157; and Louis Krasno, 33–35, 154; and Krebiozen, "fair test" of, 73, 101–106, 109–13, 130; and Krebiozen, first experiments with, 33–34; and Krebiozen fraud trial, 2, 14, 139–46, 151–53; and Krebiozen interstate shipping ban, 117–19, 123–24, 134, 139, 152; and Krebiozen legislative hearings, 12–13, 72–76, 81–83, 103, 155; and Krebiozen patients, 33–35, 39–41, 113, 116–20; and Krebiozen Research Foundation, 43, 87, 99–100, 108; and *Krebiozen: Thirteen Years of Bitter Controversy*, 137; labor unions' support of, 98–99; and Roland Libonati, 65, 67, 70–72, 89, 99, 108; and Diane Lindstrom, 116; and lipopolysaccharide C, 100, 112, 151; and Park Livingston, 36, 50–51, 71–72, 99; and Jack Mabley, 114, 161; and Catherine Manning, 161; and Medical Center Commission (Chicago), 52; and Josiah J. Moore, 33, 50, 69–70, 95; motivations of, 152–55, 161–62; and National Advisory Cancer Council, 32, 44; and NCI, 13, 104, 109–12, 143, 155; and Northwestern University, 21, 23, 31, 47, 53, 108; and Nuremberg Code and trials, 1, *22–23*, 137–38, 170n17; and *Observations on Krebiozen in the Management of Cancer*, 95–96; and Revilo Oliver, 96; and Stanley Olson, 36, 52–54, 57–58, 61, 94; and Louis Pasteur, 10, 70, 91, 154, 157; patronage accusations against, 71–72; and William F. P. Phillips, 34–35, 91, 95–96, 99, 144; and PHS, 101–2, 109–10; and John Pick, 35, 43–44, 94–96, 99, 110–11; and prisoner experiments, 22–23; and Miles Robinson, 134, 135, 141; and Roosevelt University, 108–9, 121, 151–52; and Allen Rutherford, 98, 99; scientific reputation of, 21, 152–57; and John Sembower, 73, 87, 134, 143–45; and Howard Shuman, 131–36; and George Stoddard libel suit, 13, 86–88, 93–94, 105–7, 113, 148; stubbornness of, 68, 154–55, 161–62; and Gloria Swanson, 13, 97–100, 157; and University of Chicago, 21, 47, 130; and U of I Board of Trustees, 50–51, 57, 60–67, 89, 107; and U of I Cole Committee, 54–58, 63, 65, 109, 155; U of I hiring of, 21–22, 53, 107; and U of I Johnson Committee, 57, 59–60; and U of I medical programs, 21–23, 51–68, 71–72, 107, 161; U of I separation from, 107–8

Ivy Cancer Leagues, 13, 100, 151, 152

Ivy Cancer Research Foundation, 100, 108, 114, 161

"J'Accuse . . . !" (Zola), 91, 93

JAMA. See Journal of the American Medical Association

James, Edmund J., 24

James, Thomas, 141

Jarrell, Randall, 20

Jenkins, Charles, 65, 67, 70

John Birch Society, 96

Johnson, Lyndon B., 14, 130, 132–33, 137, 156

Johnson, Robert, 57, 59–60

Johnson Committee. *See* University of Illinois Johnson Committee

Johnston, Wayne, 81

Jones, Boisfeuillet, 113, 118, 120, 123, 131, 133

Jones, Howard Mumford, 20

Jones, Wade, 94–95

Journal of the American Medical Association (JAMA), 45, 49, 76, 81–82, 91, 104. *See also* American Medical Association

journalism, 9–10; Durovic brothers, coverage of, 41–43, 74, 101, 137; Andrew Ivy, coverage of, 23, 74, 131, 138–39, 152–54, 157;

Krebiozen, coverage of, 39–43, 49–50, 57–61, 66, 74, 113–14, 131, 138–39, 157; U of I, coverage of, 18, 27–29, 65–66, 74, 80–81, 107. *See also names of individual journalists and publications*

K, Krebiozen—Key to Cancer? (Bailey), 90–94, 96–97. See also *Matter of Life or Death, A*

Kasson, David, 96, 98, 102

Kefauver, Estes, 112

Kefauver-Harris Amendment, 113, 156

Kelly-Nash machine (Chicago), 26, 129

Kelsey, Frances Oldham, 9, 112–13, 142

Ken-L Ration, 121–22

Kennedy, Edward, 158

Kennedy, John F., 114, 118, 132

Kennelly, Martin, 36

Kerr, Clark, 24

Kessler, Ruth, *125*, 126

Kirk, Paul, 103

Koch, William Frederick, 4, 89–90, 93, 128, 156; academic credentials of, 69–70, 158

Kositerin, 10, 30–32, 74, 154, 172n43; in Argentina, 30, 34, 73–74, 82; Illinois legislature's hearings on, 81–82; Northwestern University's tests of, 31–32, 42, 61, 74, 153

Krasno, Louis, 33–35, 154

Krebiozen, *55*; AMA investigation of, 12, 46–50, 54, 61, 91–94; and American Cancer Society, 96, 102–4, 155; "fair test" of, 2, 13, 73, 100–106, 109–14, 130; FDA investigation of, 13–14, 113, 120–28, 132, 138–40, 142, 157; fraud trial, 139–150, 156; interstate shipping ban, 13–14, 117–19, 123–24, 134, 139, 152; journalism's coverage of, 39–43, 49–50, 57–61, 66, 74, 113–14, 131, 138–39, 157; labor unions' support of, 98–99, 147, 157; legislative hearings on, 12–13, 72–76, 81–83, 103, 155;

MATTHEW C. EHRLICH is professor emeritus of journalism at the University of Illinois. He has previously published five books including *Dangerous Ideas on Campus: Sex, Conspiracy, and Academic Freedom in the Age of JFK* and *Kansas City vs. Oakland: The Bitter Sports Rivalry That Defined an Era.*

The University of Illinois Press
is a founding member of the
Association of University Presses.

———————————————————————

Composed in 11.25/13 Adobe Garamond
with Gotham display
by Kirsten Dennison
at the University of Illinois Press
Manufactured by Sheridan Books, Inc.

University of Illinois Press
1325 South Oak Street
Champaign, IL 61820-6903
www.press.uillinois.edu